i

THE SACRED SHADE – SECRETS OF CHAYA CHIKITSA AND FOREST HEALING

First Edition, 2025
ISBN 978-1-7342115-3-5

For any further information, contact: www.wellbeen.com

ACKNOWLEDGEMENTS

To Mother Earth, the eternal source of nourishment and healing.

To my Guru, Bhagawan Sri Sathya Sai Baba, whose divine presence illumines my path.

To Sadguru Sri Madhusudan Sai, with deep love and gratitude, for his constant encouragement, his call to serve others, and his vision that inspires me to honor nature's wisdom in the journey of healing.

To my father, whose unwavering guidance strengthens me.

To my loving and kind family, for always encouraging me, for embracing the natural ways of nourishment, and for patiently being pulled into countless botanical and herbal gardens along the way.

And above all, to the innate intelligence of the Universe, for gifting humanity with plants, herbs, and superfoods—sacred companions in our well-being.

For me, gratitude is not merely an attitude, but the very rhythm and truth of the Universe.

PREFACE

In every ancient culture, trees were not merely seen as resources for wood, fruit, or shelter—they were honored as living beings, guardians of wisdom, and vessels of healing. Whether in Indian forests, African plains, or Celtic groves, humanity has always looked at trees as living temples. Their shade, fruits, flowers, and aura carry healing for body, mind, and spirit. In the Vedic tradition, Ayurveda and Siddhas recognized them as carriers of prāṇa (life force), whose shade and presence could restore balance to body, mind, and spirit. This subtle art of healing through the protective aura of trees is known as Chhaya Chikitsa—the therapy of shade.

This book is a humble attempt to reawaken that forgotten wisdom. At a time when modern life is moving us further from nature, Chhaya Chikitsa reminds us that healing does not always come in capsules, syrups, or even herbal decoctions—it can also come through something as simple, profound, and accessible as sitting quietly under a sacred tree.

Through stories, traditional healing insights, classical references, and practical guidance, this book explores how trees like Peepal, Neem, Banyan, Kadamba, Ashoka, and Tulsi continue to heal us silently. Each tree has a unique aura, a subtle vibration that resonates with our inner being—cooling anger, calming fear, uplifting sadness, or strengthening the heart. May these pages invite you to step into the shade with reverence, to breathe deeply under the canopy of leaves, and to remember that the Earth herself is the first physician. To sit under a tree is not merely rest—it is communion, it is therapy, it is prayer.

I offer this work as a bridge between the ancient forests of wisdom and the seekers of today who long for natural, holistic, and soulful healing. With gratitude to the sages, seers, and trees who have preserved this knowledge, I welcome you into the healing shade.

— *Rev. Dr. Gauri M. Relan*

CONTENTS

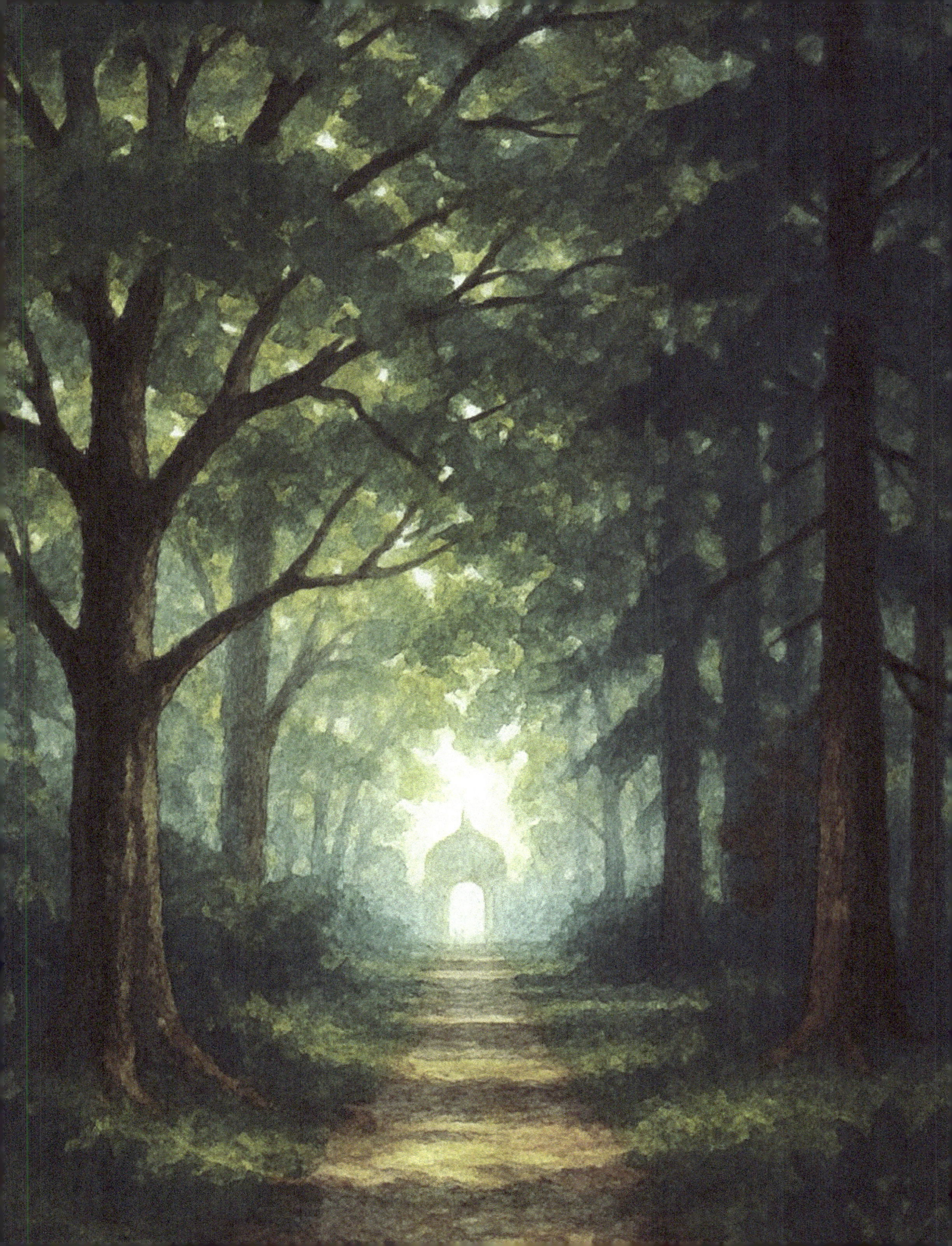

"When we rest beneath a tree's shade
or walk slowly through the forest, we are entering the same temple
through two doors — one carved by ancient wisdom, the other illuminated
by modern science.

Chhaya Chikitsa speaks the language of prana, doshas, and sacred
memory, while Forest Therapy speaks the language of nervous system
balance, stress reduction, and immunity.

Yet both reveal the same truth: that the shade of trees is living medicine,
silently cooling the mind, softening the heart, and reminding us of our
belonging to the greater web of life."

INTRODUCTION

Chhāyā Chikitsā (shade therapy) and modern forest therapy (Shinrin-yoku / forest bathing) are two expressions of the same timeless wisdom — nature heals through presence, shade, and subtle vibration. They complement and enrich each other beautifully!

HOW THEY GO HAND IN HAND

1. Healing through Shade & Light

- Chhāyā Chikitsā emphasizes sitting or resting in the shade of specific trees for balance of doshas and mental cooling.
- Forest Therapy immerses a person in the shifting play of light and shadow in the forest canopy, regulating mood and stress.

2. Nervous System Reset

- Both slow down the sympathetic "fight or flight" mode.
- The filtered light of shade lowers cortisol, balances heart rate, and creates deep relaxation.

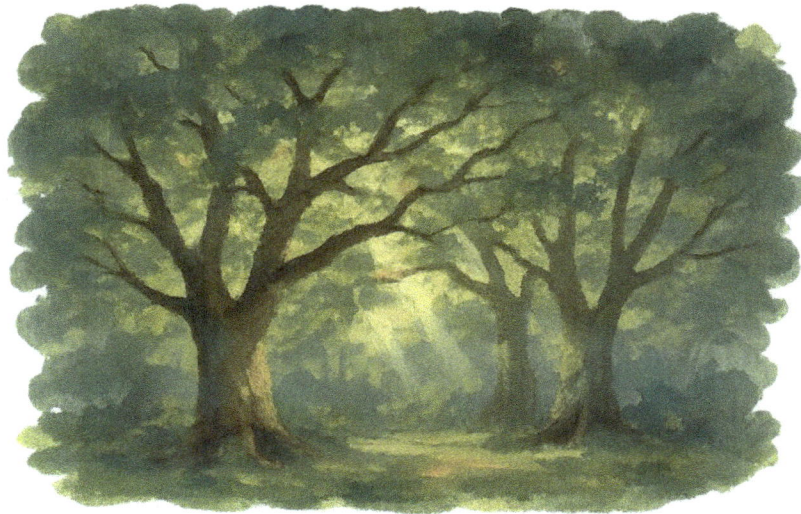

3. Subtle Energy Absorption

- Ayurveda sees shade as infused with prāṇa of the tree — Banyan gives stability, Neem purifies, Peepal uplifts consciousness.
- Forest therapy research shows phytoncides (plant aerosols) reduce anxiety, depression, and strengthen immunity.

4. Cooling the Mind's Fire

- Chhāyā chikitsā balances pitta in the mind: anger, irritation, overthinking.
- Forest therapy gives similar results, with studies showing reduced rumination and greater emotional clarity.

5. Sense of Belonging & Wholeness

- Chhāyā chikitsā invokes ancestral memory — people sitting under sacred trees for satsang, meditation, or healing.
- Forest therapy reconnects one to the ecological self — feeling part of the living Earth community.

6. Meditation without Effort

- In both practices, healing happens just by being — no force, no intense techniques.
- The shade and the forest do the work silently, drawing the mind inward into balance and calm.

In short: Chhāyā Chikitsā is like the sacred, Vedic root of what we now call Forest Therapy.

One is the traditional spiritual lens, the other a modern scientific lens — but both agree that shade, trees, and forests are medicine for the mind.

THE INNER WAR

A Poem of Senses, Soul, and Self-Mastery

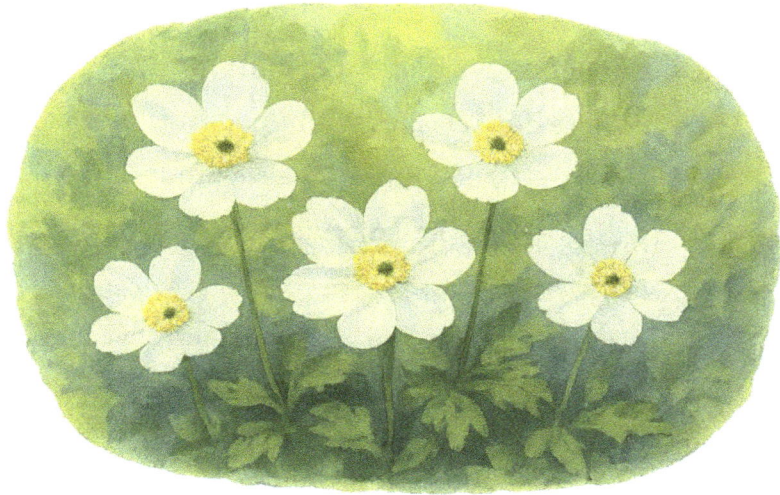

Five brave warriors ride within,
Through forest deep of thought and grin.
Sight, sound, taste, touch and
Smell that clings to things too much.

Yudhishthira walks the path of truth,
Bhima guards the fire of youth.
Arjuna seeks with focused eye,
While Nakula breathes beauty's sigh.
Sahadeva hears the silent tone—
The wisdom whispered when alone.

These are not just kings of lore,
But senses five at spirit's door.
Dragged from palace, pushed to pain,
To cleanse the mind in exile's rain.

The forest is no place of fear,
It's where the inner soul draws near.
For in the quiet, stripped of role,
The senses bow before the soul.

And on the field of doubt and storm,
Where duty clashes with the norm,
The mind—like Arjun—kneels, confused,
By life's great war, so bruised, accused.

But Krishna speaks from heart's deep cave,
"Act, dear child, be strong, be brave.
Let Karma be your outer hand,
Serve the world, but understand...

Let Bhakti be your beating flame,
Love all things without a name.
And when the mind grows clear and wise,
Let wisdom lift the final guise."

Thus, the chariot moves ahead,
Not by ego, not by dread.
But by a Self that's vast and still,
Beyond the senses, mind, and will.

So when you feel the battle start—
Confusion tearing at your heart—
Remember this: the war's within,
And victory lies where you begin.

Love and light

"When the world was young,
temples had no walls.

They were groves
of trees."

THE FORGOTTEN ART OF HEALING BY SHADE (CHHAYA)

Before the rise of modern medicine, before the written word, human beings turned to the trees. They were the first teachers, the first protectors, the first healers. We rested under their branches when weary, we prayed in their groves when lost, and we listened to their silence when searching for wisdom. This quiet communion was not superstition — it was a subtle science. The ancients called it Chhāyā Chikitsā (छाया चिकित्सा), the healing art of shade therapy.

WHAT IS CHHAYA CHIKITSA?

Chaya isn't merely a patch of shadow that stops light; it's the field of influence that extends beyond the visible — an energetic halo, an imprint, a subtle climate that reshapes what happens inside it.

- **Chhāyā** = the living shade — a non-visible field of influence that shelters, cools, and alters inner weather. It's simultaneously place and presence: an energetic aura that invites
- **Chikitsā** = therapy, treatment, healing.

It is the practice of receiving healing by simply being in the shade of trees — sitting, meditating, breathing, or resting beneath them to absorb their prana (life force), fragrance, and vibrational field.

In this art, medicine is not swallowed or applied. Medicine is received through presence.

WHY TREES HEAL BEYOND HERBS

Ayurveda recognizes that plants have two powers:

1. **Dravyaguna (material healing)**: their roots, bark, leaves, fruits, and flowers as medicines.
2. **Prabhava (subtle influence)**: their unseen vibrations, fragrances, and shade as therapy.

While modern herbalism remembers the first, the second has been almost forgotten. Yet it is this second power — the living aura of the tree — that nourishes the human heart and soul.

SACRED GROVES – NATURE'S FIRST HOSPITALS

Long before clinics, people knew where to go when they needed healing. They went to the forest.

- Temple trees like Peepal, Neem, and Banyan were planted not only for ritual, but for their shade and energy.
- Sacred groves were living pharmacies — cooling, cleansing, stabilizing body and mind.
- Hermitages were always surrounded by trees, because sages knew that wisdom ripens only in green silence.

Modern forest therapy and shinrin-yoku (forest bathing) are rediscoveries of this ancient truth: when we step into nature's shade, we step back into wholeness.

THE ESSENCE OF SHADE HEALING

In Chhāyā Chikitsā, the tree does not give you anything new. It reminds you of what you already are — whole, calm, connected.

- The shade cools the body and calms fiery Pitta.
- The fragrance uplifts the mind, clearing the heaviness of Kapha.

- The vibrations balance Vata, steadying scattered thoughts.
- The aura strengthens the spirit, reconnecting us with stillness.

A LOST ART, A LIVING INVITATION

Today, we live in houses of concrete and glass, forgetting that the shade of a single tree can do what no machine can. It can reset our nervous system, clear our breath, cool our anger, soften our sorrow, and rekindle our inner light.

Chhāyā Chikitsā is not a practice to be learned; it is a relationship to be remembered.

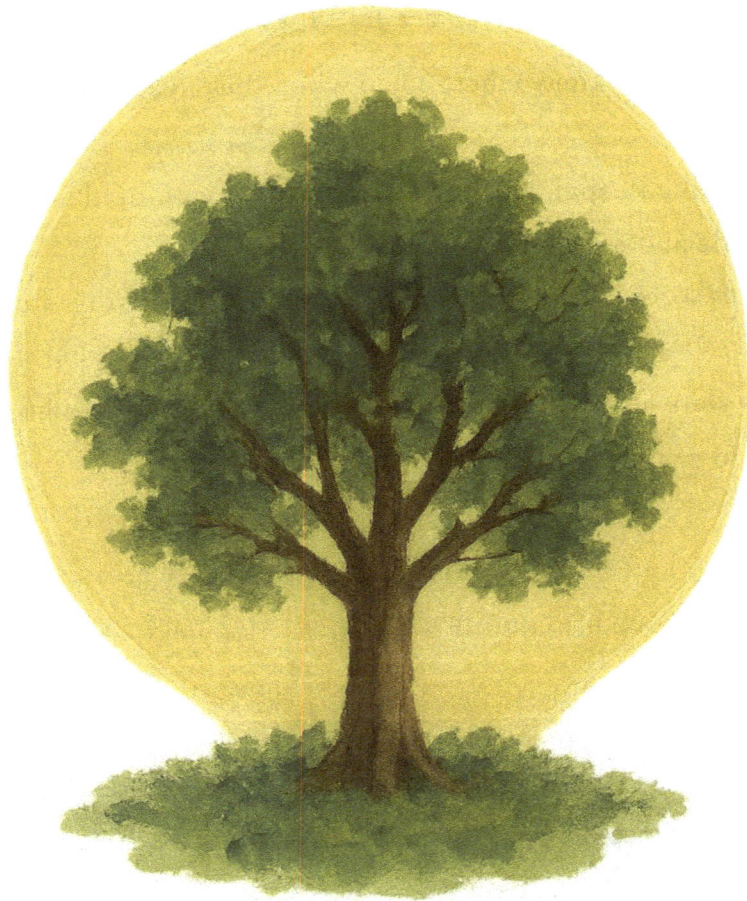

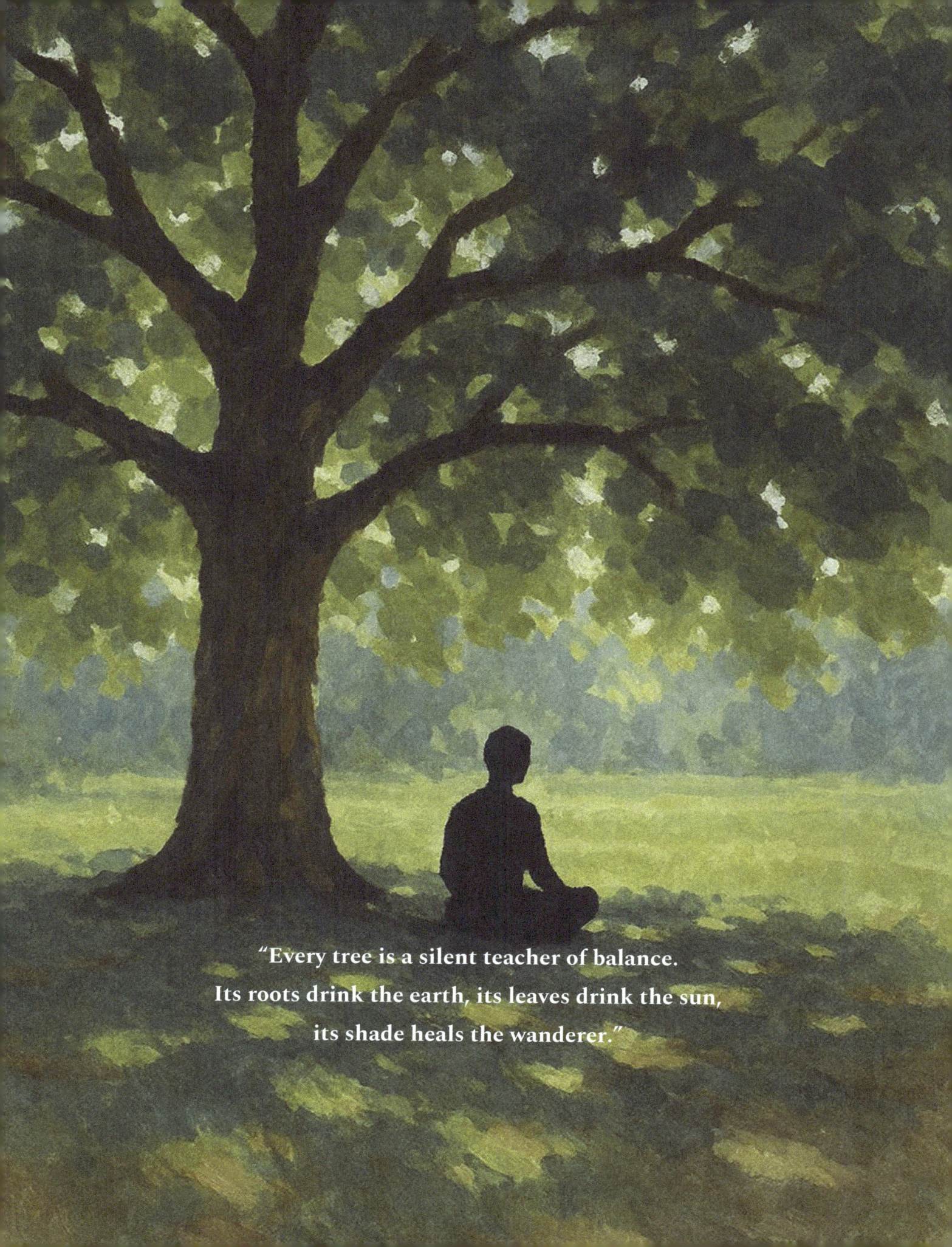

"Every tree is a silent teacher of balance.
Its roots drink the earth, its leaves drink the sun,
its shade heals the wanderer."

THE SCIENCE OF TREE PRESENCE

The ancients never separated medicine from the environment. To them, the air you breathe, the land you live upon, the shade you rest in, and even the season of the year were part of health.

Ayurveda and traditional sciences preserved this truth: a tree does not only heal through what it gives materially, but through what it radiates invisibly.

TWO DIMENSIONS OF HEALING

1. Dravyaguna (Material Properties)

- Tangible aspects like bark, roots, fruits, leaves.
- These treat the body through herbs, decoctions, and oils.

2. Prabhava (Subtle Influence)

- The vibrational, unseen quality of the tree.
- This is absorbed by simply sitting in its shade, breathing its air, entering its aura.

Thus, Chhāyā Chikitsā works primarily through Prabhava — the silent influence that reshapes our energy and emotions.

A LIVING SANCTUARY

To sit beneath a tree is to step into a living sanctuary where medicine is not prescribed but silently absorbed.

THE TREE'S SUBTLE MEDICINES

Modern science now confirms what the sages intuited — trees release phytoncides (natural aromatic compounds) that lower stress hormones and increase immune activity.

Sukshma Prabhava (subtle effect)

The aura of the tree interacts with human manovaha srotas (mental channels). Sitting under Neem cools agitation, while Kadamba sparks joy.

Gandha & Prāṇa Shakti (fragrance & oxygen)

Aroma molecules and oxygen-rich air beneath trees change mood chemistry and boost vitality.

Filtered Light (Tejas absorption)

Leaves soften harsh sunlight, calming fiery Pitta and steadying the nervous system.

Earthing through Shade

Barefoot contact with soil beneath trees grounds electromagnetic imbalance, harmonizing body rhythms.

CLASSICAL REFERENCES

Charaka Samhita & Sushruta Samhita

- Speak of desha (place), kāla (time), vayu (air), and vanaspati (vegetation) as health factors. Healing is not only through ingestion, but also through samsparsha (contact).

Raja Nighantu & Brihat Samhita

- Mention kalpavriksha and punya-vriksha (sacred trees) that bless with wellness when one simply rests in their shade.

Vriksha Ayurveda (Surapala, 10th c.)

- Advises planting sacred trees in homes, temples, and hermitages because their shade purifies the air and strengthens the mind.

HEALING THROUGH DOSHA BALANCE

Each tree has a dosha-balancing signature. By choosing the right tree, one chooses the right medicine.

Vata (air-ether): Restless minds soften under Ashoka, Kadamba, or Peepal.

Pitta (fire-water): Anger and inflammation cool under Neem, Bilva, or Banyan.

Kapha (earth-water): Heaviness and stagnation lighten under Tulsi, Arjuna, or Mango.

ECHOES IN MODERN SCIENCE

What Ayurveda called Prabhava, modern science calls biophilia — the natural healing that comes when humans reunite with green life.

Forest Bathing (Shinrin-yoku, Japan): Spending time under trees lowers cortisol, improves sleep, and boosts immunity.

Aromatherapy Science: Volatile oils released by trees act on the limbic system, calming emotions.

Light Therapy: Shade's filtering of UV reduces oxidative stress while still providing healthy wavelengths.

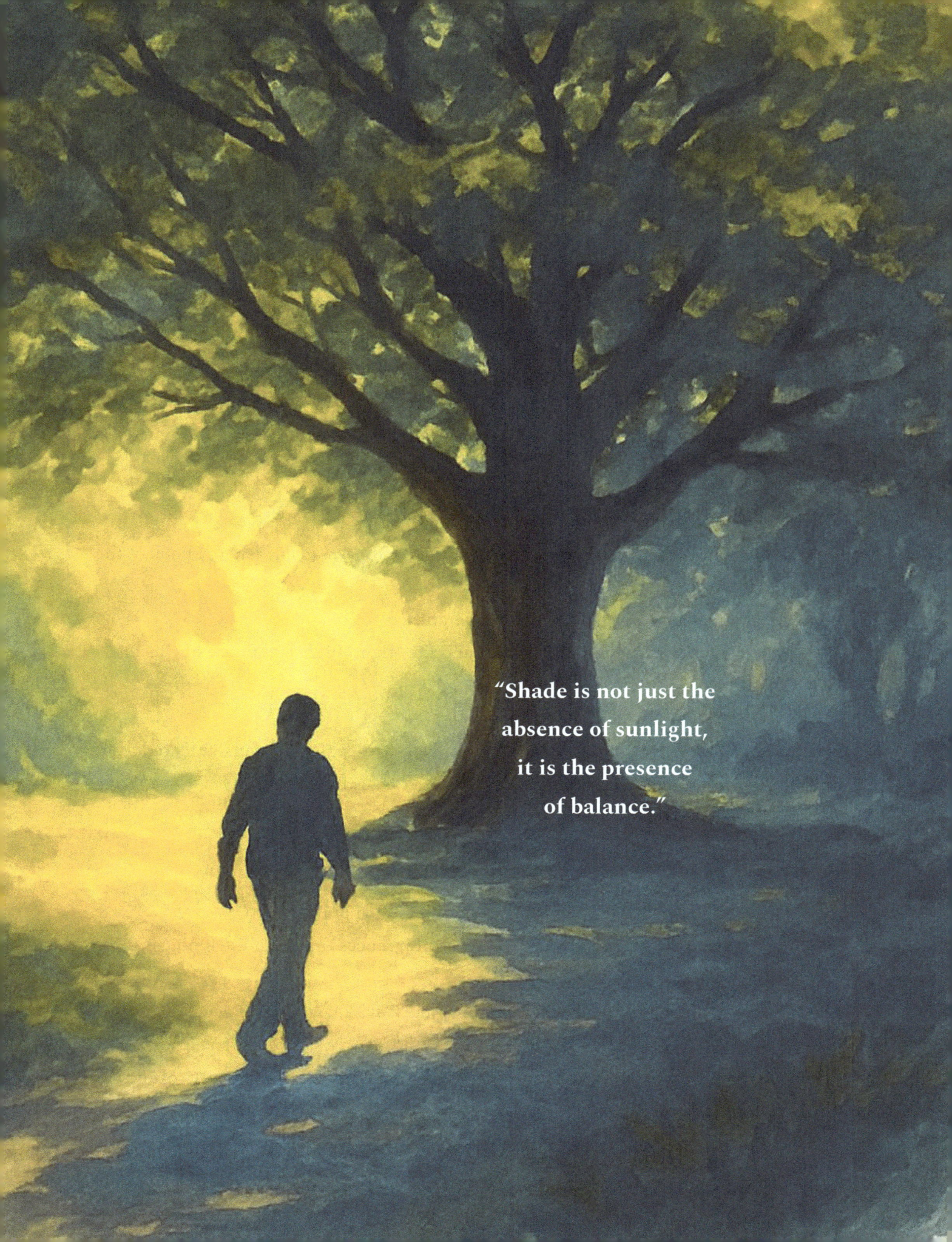

"Shade is not just the
absence of sunlight,
it is the presence
of balance."

HOW TREE SHADE HEALS

When you step under the canopy of a tree, something subtle begins to shift. The breath changes, the heartbeat softens, and the chatter of the mind finds a slower rhythm. Ayurveda teaches that this transformation is not coincidence—it is the medicine of shade.

THE FIRST ENCOUNTER: ENTERING THE CANOPY

- As you approach, your body crosses into the prabhā-mandala (energy field) of the tree.
- Heat and glare soften, your skin temperature cools.
- The nervous system registers safety, and the "fight–flight" response begins to dissolve.

Science lens: Air temperature under a tree can be 2–5°C cooler. This instantly reduces the body's stress load and calms Pitta (heat–fire).

BREATH OF LIFE: OXYGEN & AROMAS

- Trees exhale what we need most: oxygen rich with prāṇa shakti.
- Many also release sattvic aromas—subtle fragrances that calm the limbic brain.

Experience: Sitting beneath Neem clears the mind, Tulsi invigorates, Peepal deepens breath.

Science lens: Phytoncides and terpenes strengthen immunity, lowering cortisol and inflammation.

MIND IN STILLNESS: THE SHADE EFFECT

- The dappled light under leaves harmonizes tejas (inner radiance).
- This balances the pineal gland, improves circadian rhythm, and steadies wandering thoughts.

Experience: Close your eyes under Ashoka or Banyan—notice how the mind naturally turns inward.

Science lens: Gentle light stimulates serotonin, improving mood and mental clarity.

EARTHING AND GROUNDING

- The soil under trees carries electrical balance—negatively charged ions that neutralize stress energy in the body.
- By sitting or standing barefoot, one absorbs this grounding vibration.

Experience: Heaviness in the chest or anxious flutter eases after 20 minutes barefoot beneath a Mango tree.

Science lens: Grounding reduces oxidative stress and stabilizes heart rhythms.

EMOTIONAL MEDICINE

Every tree has an emotional rasa (flavor):

- **Banyan:** Nurturing, safety, continuity.
- **Neem:** Detachment, clarity, purification.
- **Ashoka:** Joy, release from grief.
- **Tulsi:** Devotion, spiritual focus.

Spending time under these trees is a therapy for the manas (mind) and hridaya (heart) as much as for the body.

THE SILENT DIALOGUE

Traditional healing says that human beings and trees are in a constant exchange:

- We exhale carbon dioxide → trees inhale.
- Trees exhale oxygen → we inhale.
- This is not just chemistry—it is prāṇic companionship, a dialogue of life.

When you sit under a tree, you re-enter this sacred cycle consciously.

A SIMPLE PRACTICE

1. Find a tree that draws you—let intuition guide you.
2. Sit quietly beneath it, feet touching the soil.
3. Take 9 slow breaths, imagining you are inhaling its exhale.
4. Place your palms on the earth, release any heavy thought or worry into the ground.
5. Close your eyes for 10–20 minutes, simply resting.

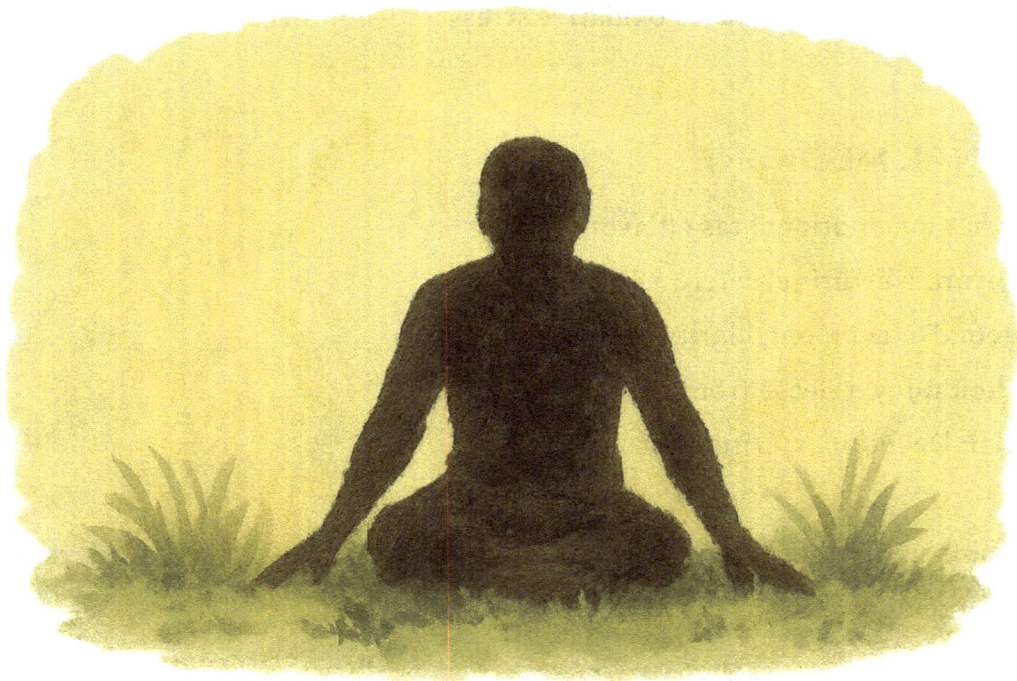

JOURNALING PROMPT

What shifted in my body, mind, and emotions after sitting in the shade?

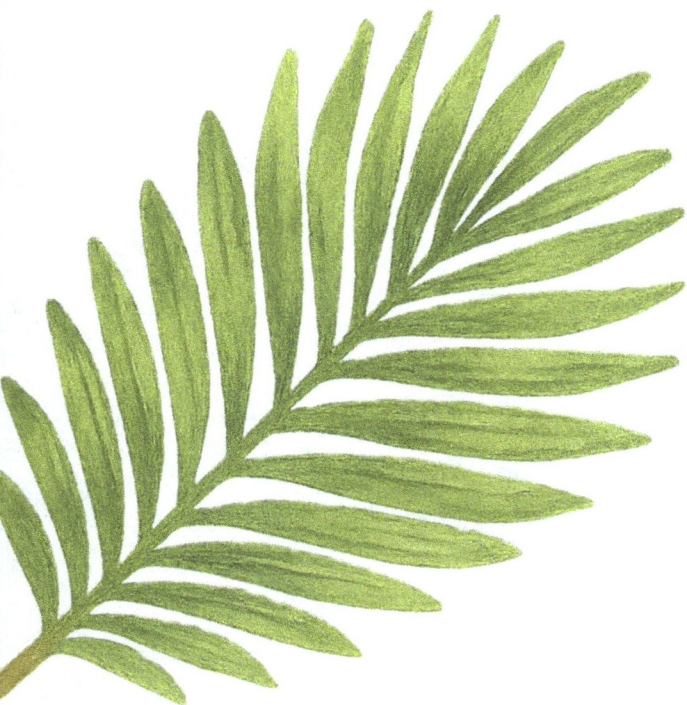

_____

_____

_____

_____

_____

_____

_____

"Every tree has a voice.
Some whisper of joy,
some sing of wisdom,
some stand in silence
holding eternity."

SACRED TREES & THEIR HEALING PERSONALITIES

Ayurveda and world traditions regard trees as living medicines—not only for their leaves, bark, and roots, but for their presence. Each tree carries a distinct bhāva (emotional quality) and dosha-balancing signature.

PEEPAL (FICUS RELIGIOSA) – THE BREATH OF INFINITY

Healing Personality: Expansive, uplifting, deeply spiritual.

Dosha Effect: Balances Vata by calming the restless mind.

Sacred Story: Under a Peepal, the Buddha attained enlightenment—its shade still resonates with silence and awakening.

Healing Vibe: Sit beneath to feel connected to the infinite, especially during dawn.

NEEM (AZADIRACHTA INDICA) – THE GREAT PURIFIER

Healing Personality: Cooling, clarifying, detached.

Dosha Effect: Pacifies fiery Pitta, detoxifies blood and emotions.

Sacred Story: Called Arista ("reliever of all disease"), Neem is considered a goddess tree, offering protection from both visible and invisible poisons.

Healing Vibe: Best for releasing anger, cooling inflammation—both in body and mind.

ASHOKA (SARACA ASOCA) – THE TREE OF JOY

Healing Personality: Joy-bringer, light-hearted, reliever of sorrow.

Dosha Effect: Soothes Pitta (emotions of grief, burning heart).

Sacred Story: Sita stayed under Ashoka trees in Lanka. The tree's name literally means "without sorrow."

Healing Vibe: Sit beneath Ashoka when carrying grief, to lighten the heart.

BANYAN (FICUS BENGHALENSIS) – THE ETERNAL SHELTER

Healing Personality: Protective, grounding, stabilizing.

Dosha Effect: Balances Vata and Kapha by offering stillness and safety.

Sacred Story: Called Vata Vriksha, its endless aerial roots symbolize continuity of life. Often associated with Yama (God of time), representing endurance.

Healing Vibe: Meditate under Banyan for grounding, security, and long life.

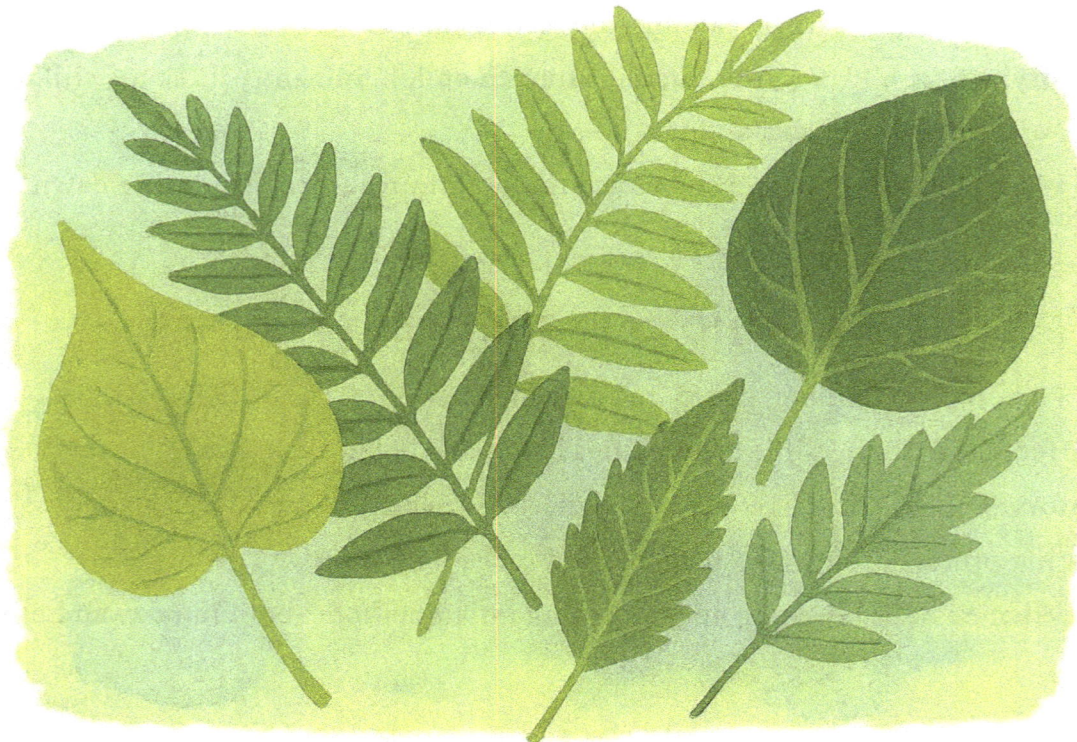

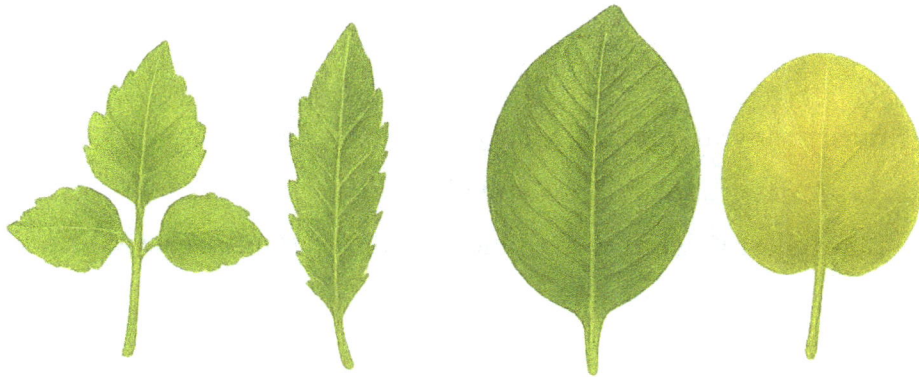

TULSI (OCIMUM SANCTUM) – THE HOLY PROTECTOR

Healing Personality: Devotional, purifying, energizing.

Dosha Effect: Clears Kapha stagnation and uplifts Vata dullness.

Sacred Story: Beloved of Vishnu, Tulsi is worshiped in courtyards as a living goddess.

Healing Vibe: Sit near Tulsi to awaken devotion, clarity, and protection.

ARJUNA (TERMINALIA ARJUNA) – GUARDIAN OF THE HEART

Healing Personality: Strong, steady, warrior-like.

Dosha Effect: Strengthens the heart, balancing Kapha heaviness.

Sacred Story: Named after the Mahabharata hero Arjuna, known for courage and loyalty.

Healing Vibe: A companion for those facing fear, stress, or matters of the heart.

COCONUT (COCOS NUCIFERA) – THE TREE OF BLESSINGS

Healing Personality: Nourishing, giving, cooling.

Dosha Effect: Balances Pitta heat, hydrates and refreshes.

Sacred Story: Considered auspicious, the coconut is offered in every ritual as a symbol of surrender and purity.

Healing Vibe: Sit beneath a coconut palm for cooling thoughts, letting go, and renewal.

KADAMBA (NEOLAMARCKIA CADAMBA) – THE TREE OF DIVINE PLAY

Healing Personality: Joyful, romantic, playful.

Dosha Effect: Lifts Vata sadness and Kapha heaviness.

Sacred Story: Beloved of Krishna, who danced under Kadamba groves with the gopīs.

Healing Vibe: Best for creativity, love, and childlike joy.

HOW TO RELATE TO TREE PERSONALITIES

- Visit different trees at different times of day.
- Observe your mood shift—do you feel lighter, calmer, or more grounded?
- Keep a tree journal to note emotional changes.

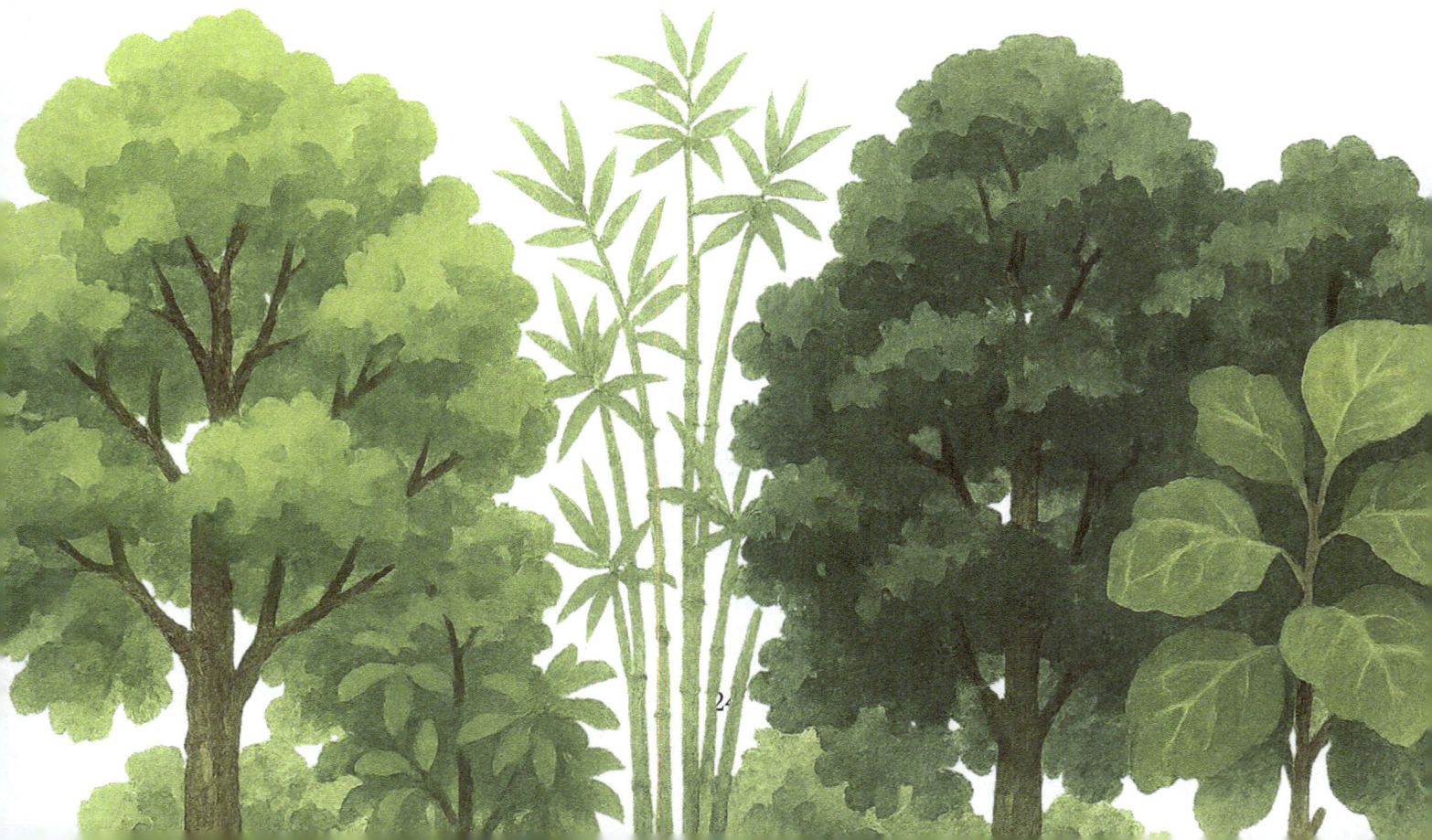

"Sit under a tree for a while,
and you will find the medicine of silence."

NADI PRIKSA – THE ART OF PULSE DIAGNOSIS

WHAT IT MEANS

Nāḍī Prikṣā (Sanskrit: nāḍī = pulse/channel, parīkṣā = examination) is an ancient Ayurvedic diagnostic technique where a Vaidya (Ayurvedic physician) reads the pulse at the wrist to understand the balance of the three doshas—Vata, Pitta, and Kapha—as well as deeper imbalances in the body and mind.

It is considered both a science and an art, requiring sensitivity, intuition, and years of practice.

WHERE IT IS MEASURED

The pulse is usually examined on the radial artery at the wrist, just below the thumb.

The physician places three fingers:
- Index finger = Vata
- Middle finger = Pitta
- Ring finger = Kapha

Each finger feels a different dimension of the flow.

WHAT IS OBSERVED

The physician assesses not just the rate, but many subtle qualities of the pulse:

- Gati (movement): e.g., snake-like, frog-like, swan-like, each linked to a dosha.
- Tala (rhythm): steady, irregular, fast, slow.
- Tvara (speed): how quickly it beats.
- Bala (strength): weak, moderate, strong.
- Akṛti (form): the overall impression, smooth, rough, sharp, heavy.

PULSE SIGNATURES OF THE DOSHAS

- Vata Pulse: Irregular, thin, like a snake moving—quick, uneven.
- Pitta Pulse: Strong, bounding, like a frog leaping—warm and sharp.
- Kapha Pulse: Slow, steady, like a swan gliding—deep and smooth.

Often, combinations are felt, revealing dual-dosha or tri-dosha states.

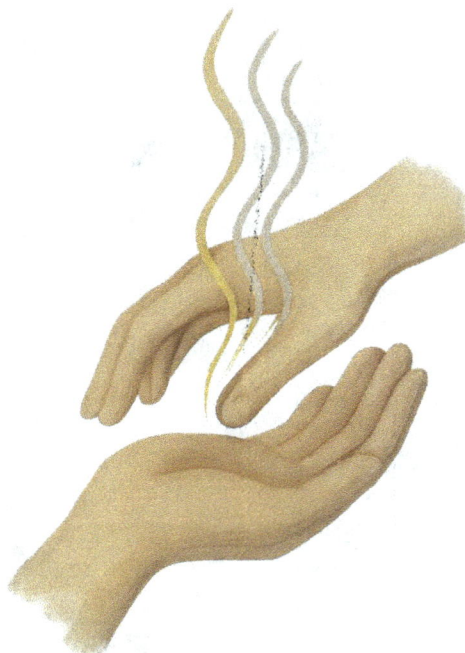

WHAT CAN BE SEEN THROUGH NADI PRIKSA

1. Prakriti (Constitution): The natural doshic makeup of a person.
2. Vikruti (Imbalance): The current disturbance in doshas.
3. Agni (Digestive Fire): Strength or weakness of metabolism.
4. Dhatus (Tissues): Condition of plasma, blood, muscle, fat, bone, marrow, and reproductive tissue.
5. Ojas (Vitality): The overall immune strength and resilience.
6. Manas (Mind): Emotional tendencies, stress levels, mental clarity.

Some masters can even detect past traumas or emotional states stored in the body.

SPIRITUAL DIMENSION

Traditional texts say that in the deepest pulse (sūkṣma nāḍī), one can feel the connection of the individual soul (jīvātman) with the cosmic soul (paramātman). Thus, pulse reading becomes not just diagnosis, but a form of listening to the life-force itself.

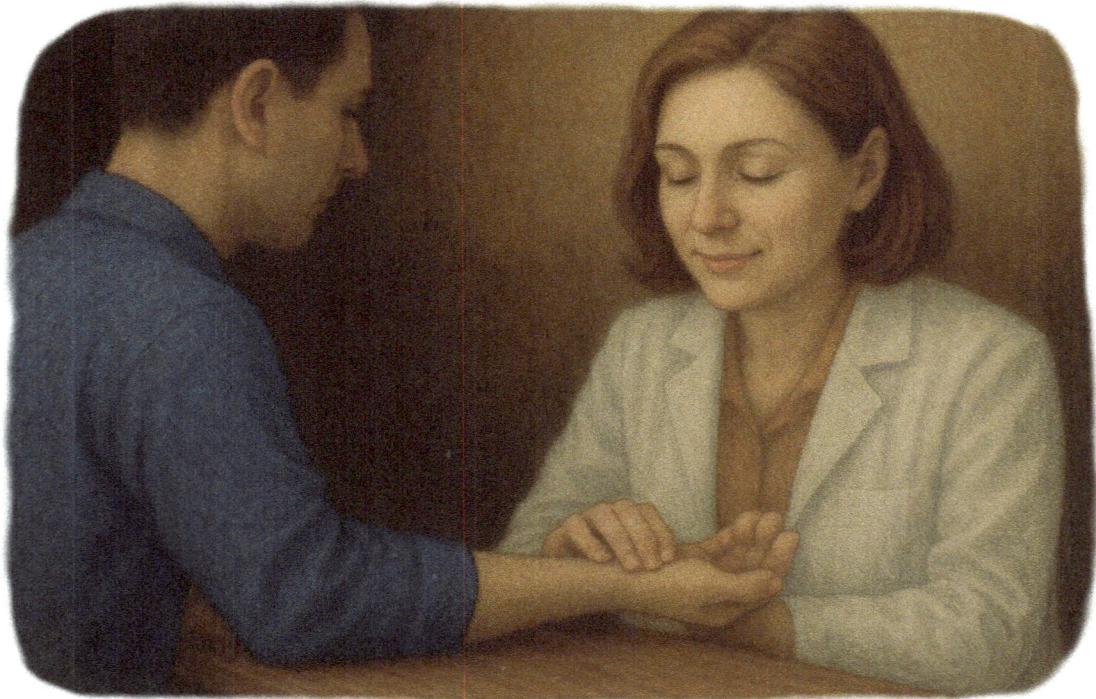

MODERN PARALLELS

Western medicine measures pulse mainly for rate and rhythm.
Ayurveda sees the pulse as a mirror of total health, integrating body, mind, and spirit.

In short: Nāḍī Prikṣa is like listening to the secret music of the body. It tells the story of balance, imbalance, and potential healing pathways.

HOW NADI PRIKSA HELPS IDENTIFY PRAKRITI & THE RIGHT HEALING TREE

1. Prakriti – Your Innate Nature

Prakriti is your natural constitution, determined by the unique balance of Vata (air/space), Pitta (fire/water), and Kapha (earth/water) within you.
Nādi Prikṣā reveals this by listening to the subtle pulse patterns that show your body's baseline tendencies.

Example:
- A Vata prakriti person → naturally creative, mobile, airy, but prone to anxiety & dryness.
- A Pitta prakriti person → sharp, focused, fiery, but prone to inflammation & irritability.
- A Kapha prakriti person → nurturing, steady, grounding, but prone to stagnation & heaviness.

Knowing your prakriti is like holding your personal energy blueprint.

2. Vikruti – Current Imbalance

Beyond your baseline nature, Nādi Prikṣa shows vikruti, i.e., where you are out of balance right now.

Example:

- A Pitta person in balance may radiate leadership and clarity.
- But when Pitta is aggravated (revealed in the pulse), it shows up as inflammation, anger, acidity → and needs cooling support.

So Nādi Prikṣa doesn't just tell who you are by nature but where you are today.

3. Trees as Dosha-Balancers (Chhāyā Chikitsā)

Each tree has dravyaguna (physical properties) and prabhāva (subtle energy qualities). By matching your prakriti/vikruti with the right tree, you restore harmony.

Vata types or imbalances (anxious, restless, ungrounded):

- Ashoka, Peepal, Kadamba – calming, grounding, soothe the mind.
- Pitta types or imbalances (angry, inflamed, overheated):
- Neem, Banyan, Bilva – cooling, anti-inflammatory, reduce excess heat.
- Kapha types or imbalances (sluggish, heavy, attached):
- Tulsi, Arjuna, Mango – uplifting, energizing, clear stagnation.

4. The Flow of Healing

- Step 1 – Nādi Prikṣa: Identify your prakriti (baseline) and vikruti (current imbalance).
- Step 2 – Tree Prescription: Select a tree whose shade qualities balance your dominant/imbalanced dosha.
- Step 3 – Chhāyā Chikitsā: Sit under that tree daily, barefoot, if possible, breathe in its prāṇa, meditate or journal.
- Step 4 – Transformation: Over time, subtle shifts happen in body, emotions, and spirit as your energies realign.

In essence: Nādi Prikṣa is the diagnosis, Prakriti is your nature, Vikruti is your imbalance, and Chhāyā Chikitsā is your personalized medicine.

DOSHA–TREE HEALING CHART (CHHĀYĀ CHIKITSĀ GUIDE)

Vata (Air + Ether)

- Nature: Creative, mobile, quick, imaginative — but prone to anxiety, dryness, restlessness.
- Imbalance signs: Overthinking, insomnia, fear, constipation, joint pain.
- Healing Trees:
  - Peepal (Ficus religiosa) – Calms the mind, deepens breath, enhances meditation. Sacred to Vishnu & Buddha.
  - Ashoka (Saraca asoca) – Relieves grief, nurtures feminine energy, balances apana vata. "Tree without sorrow."
  - Kadamba (Neolamarckia cadamba) – Uplifts mood, relieves mental heaviness, joyful aura. Sacred to Krishna's play (Lila).
- Healing Shade Effect: Grounding, calming, restoring stability to scattered prana.

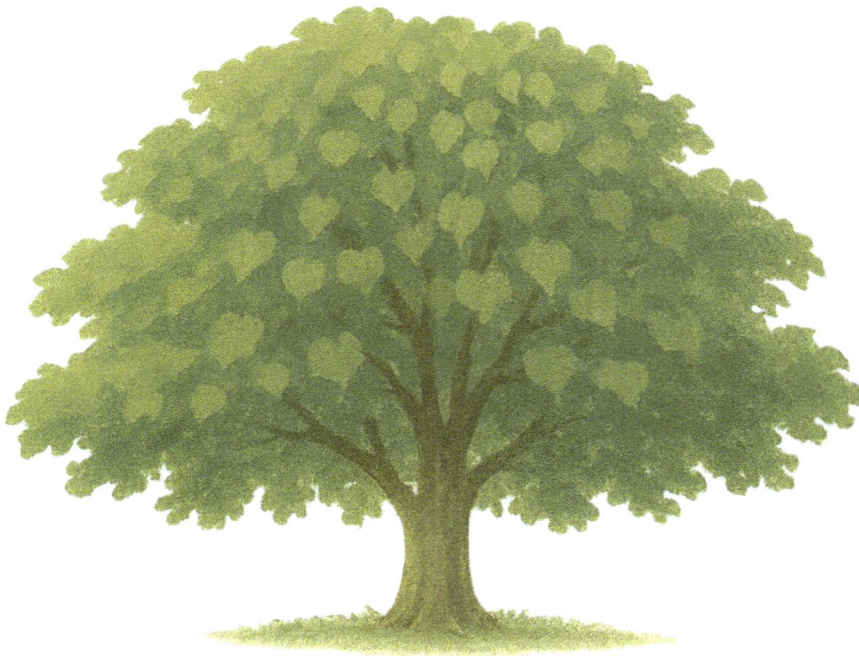

Pitta (Fire + Water)

- Nature: Intelligent, sharp, focused, transformative — but prone to anger, inflammation, heat.
- Imbalance signs: Acidity, rashes, ulcers, irritability, perfectionism.
- Healing Trees:
    - Neem (Azadirachta indica) – Cooling aura, antibacterial, reduces heat & toxins. Symbol of protection.
    - Banyan (Ficus benghalensis) – Stability, longevity, deeply cooling shade, balances intensity.
    - Bilva (Aegle marmelos) – Cools digestive fire, sacred to Shiva, clears inflammation.
- Healing Shade Effect: Cooling, pacifying, soothing fiery emotions & bodily heat.

Kapha (Earth + Water)

- Nature: Stable, nurturing, steady, compassionate — but prone to heaviness, lethargy, attachment.
- Imbalance signs: Obesity, congestion, depression, resistance to change.
- Healing Trees:
    - Tulsi (Ocimum sanctum) – Uplifts prana, clears stagnation, harmonizes emotions. Sacred to Krishna/Vishnu.
    - Arjuna (Terminalia arjuna) – Strengthens the heart, stabilizes circulation, energizes dullness.
    - Mango (Mangifera indica) – Inspires devotion, energizes, removes lethargy.
- Healing Shade Effect: Stimulating, energizing, uplifting stuck energy and emotions.

HOW TO USE THIS CHART

1. Get your Nādi Prikṣā done (or self-assess prakriti tendencies).
2. Match your dominant/imbalanced dosha to the recommended tree.
3. Daily practice: Sit/meditate under the chosen tree for 15–30 minutes.
4. Absorb the prāṇa: Breathe deeply, let the shade filter into body and mind.
5. Optional: Journal emotions or chant silently while under the tree.

Tree	Healing Shade Effect	Symbolism
Peepal (Ficus religiosa)	Calms anxiety, enhances prana, improves focus in meditation	Sacred to Vishnu, Buddha's enlightenment tree
Banyan (Ficus benghalensis)	Gives grounding, strength, longevity	Tree of stability, fertility
Neem (Azadirachta indica)	Antimicrobial aura, purifies air and energy	Symbol of protection, immunity
Kadamba (Neolamarckia cadamba)	Fills heart with joy, devotion, lightness	Krishna's tree of play (Lila), bliss
Ashoka (Saraca asoca)	Eases grief, nurtures feminine energy	"Without sorrow" – brings emotional relief
Tulsi (Ocimum sanctum)	Purifies atmosphere, harmonizes emotions	Sacred to Vishnu/Krishna, devotion and clarity

This chart becomes a sample of a living prescription — your prakriti guides the tree, and the tree restores your balance.

"In every culture,
the forest was the first pharmacy,
the river the first medicine,
the mountain the first temple.

Healing has always been a
dialogue with nature."

THE LIVING SANCTUARIES OF HEALING

From the earliest times, human beings have turned to forests, rivers, mountains, and gardens not merely as sources of survival but as sanctuaries of renewal. Modern science now validates what ancient traditions always practiced—that nature is medicine. Forests lower stress hormones, strengthen immunity, calm the heart, and rewire the brain toward peace. Ancient healing cultures knew this intuitively, creating sanctuaries where body, mind, and spirit could find restoration.

This chapter bridges science and tradition, showing how sanctuaries of healing have existed across civilizations and how they continue to inspire us today.

NATURAL SANCTUARIES: EARTH'S HEALING GROVES

Sacred Groves

- India, Africa, Europe: forests preserved as sacred spaces where cutting a tree was taboo.
- India's Devrais and Sarna Sthal: still alive in tribal regions, functioning as ecological sanctuaries and spiritual pharmacies.
- These groves balanced ecosystems, provided herbs, and offered communities a living temple of nature.

Mountains & Springs

- Himalayas: where rishis meditated, drawing longevity and clarity from snow-fed rivers and mountain air.
- Greek Mount Olympus: the seat of the gods, where seekers went on vision quests.
- Lourdes, France: waters blessed with miraculous cures.
- Native American hot springs: steaming waters for purification and rebirth.

Healing Forests & Gardens

- Shinrin-yoku (Japan): "forest bathing," proven to reduce cortisol and balance the nervous system.
- Persian gardens (pairidaeza): designed to embody harmony of the four elements—earth, water, air, and fire.
- European monastic gardens: cultivated with lavender, sage, rosemary, chamomile—herbs that healed both body and soul.

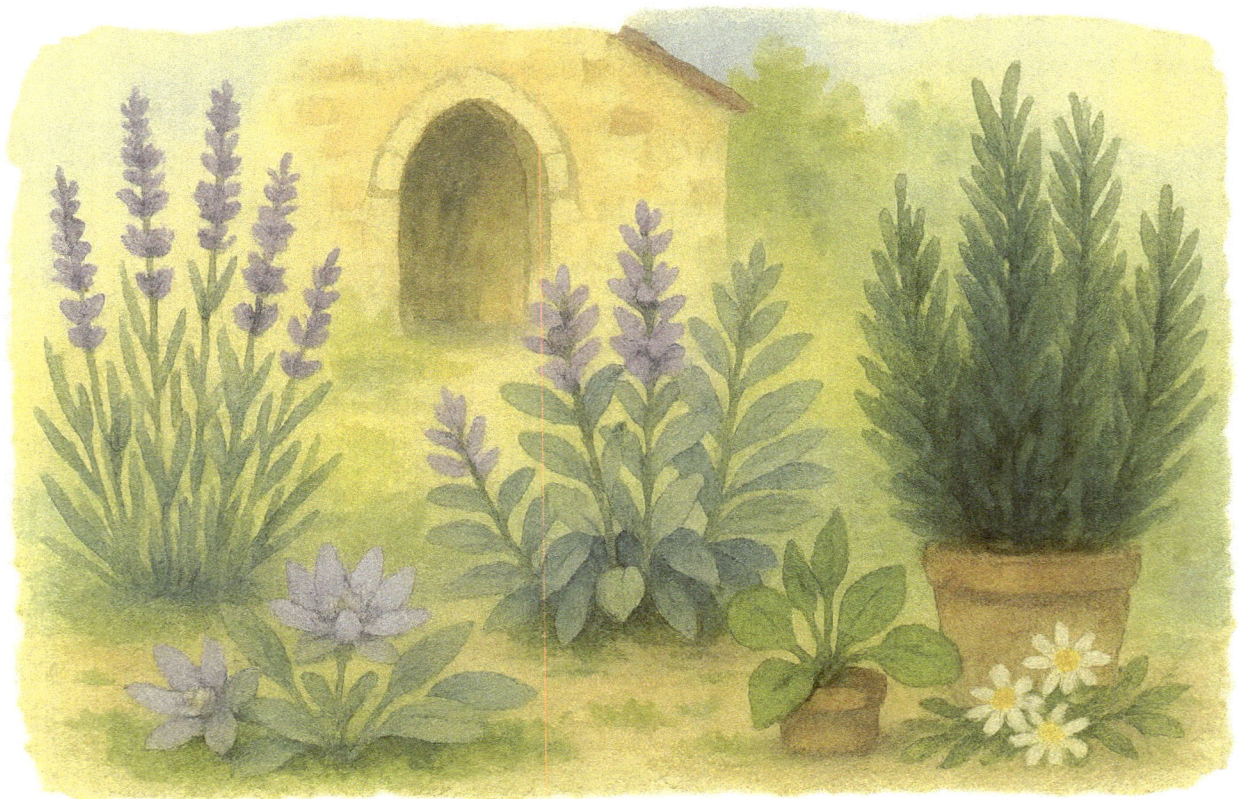

SPIRITUAL SANCTUARIES: WHEN NATURE MEETS SPIRIT

Ayurvedic Ashrams (India)

Forest hermitages where sages blended yoga, meditation, and herbal remedies, creating complete healing ecosystems. Many such ashrams still thrive today.

Greek Asclepeia (Greece)

Temples dedicated to Asclepius, god of healing. Patients slept in sacred chambers, receiving cures through dreams, rituals, and nature-inspired therapies.

Christian Monastic Sanctuaries (Europe)

Abbeys and monasteries became hospitals, where prayer, herbalism, and rest in gardens restored health.

Indigenous Healing Circles

Across the Americas, Africa, and Oceania: sweat lodges, sacred fires, and medicine wheels. These practices harmonized humans with earth, ancestors, and spirit.

MODERN HEALING SANCTUARIES

Wellness Retreats in Nature

- Forest therapy centers in Scandinavia and Japan.
- Ayurvedic wellness retreats in Kerala and Sri Lanka.
- Yoga ashrams around the world offering healing through practice, diet, and silence.

Eco-Spiritual Spaces

- Findhorn (Scotland): a community woven around conscious co-existence with nature.
- Auroville (India): an experimental city where human unity and ecological healing go hand in hand.

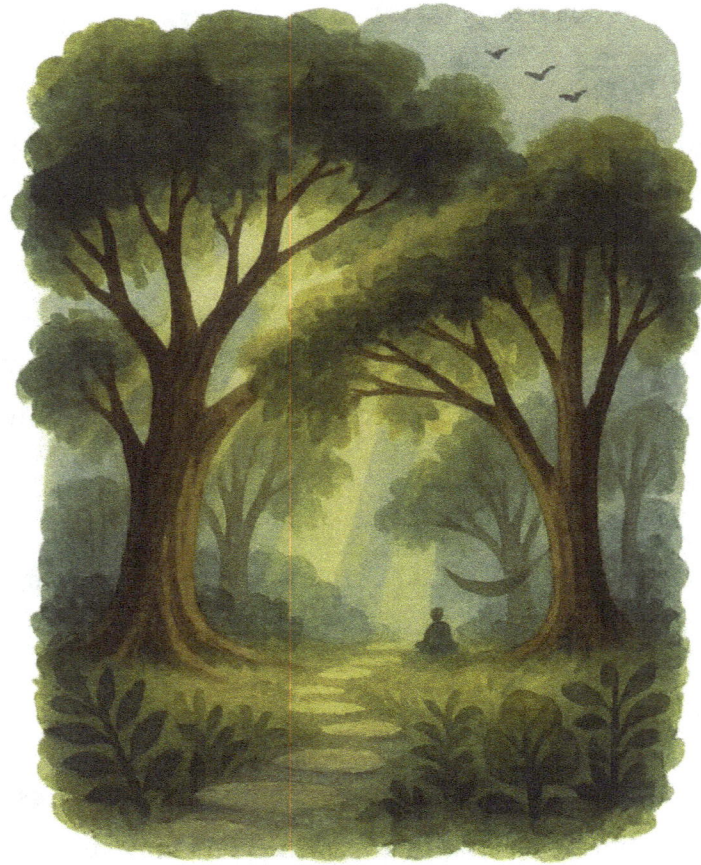

Medical-Nature Integration

- Sanatoriums in the Alps: where crisp air and mountain forests were prescribed for tuberculosis patients.
- Biophilic hospitals (Singapore, US): blending gardens, natural light, and forest courtyards into healing architecture.

From the sacred groves of India to Japanese forest paths, from Greek temples of healing dreams to modern biophilic hospitals, humanity has always sought healing sanctuaries where nature and spirit meet.

They remind us that true health is not just the absence of disease, but the presence of wholeness—a harmony of body, mind, community, and earth.

"The forest is not merely a place to visit—
it is a living pharmacy,
a sanctuary where the body
remembers balance."

THE SCIENCE OF FOREST HEALING

NATURE MEETS NEUROSCIENCE

Forests are no longer only the backdrop of myth and meditation—they are now at the frontier of medical science. Research in Japan, Europe, and the United States confirms that forests act as living laboratories of health, altering our biochemistry, balancing our physiology, and soothing our minds.

This chapter explores how trees heal us through measurable pathways—bridging ancient wisdom with modern science.

LOWER STRESS HORMONES: CORTISOL REDUCTION

Fact: Japanese studies on Shinrin-yoku ("forest bathing") reveal that immersion in forests dramatically lowers cortisol, the body's primary stress hormone.

Mechanism:
- Gentle sounds of leaves and birdsong reset the nervous system.
- Green wavelengths of light calm the visual cortex.
- Phytoncides—essential oils released by trees—act like aromatherapy, soothing the sympathetic ("fight or flight") response.

IMMUNE SYSTEM BOOST: PHYTONCIDES AND NK CELLS

Fact: Trees such as pine, cedar, and oak release volatile organic compounds called phytoncides, which increase the activity of natural killer (NK) cells in humans. NK cells are vital immune defenders against infections and even cancer.

Study Highlight: In 2009, Japanese researcher Qing Li found that a 2-day trip to a forest raised NK cell activity significantly, and the effect lasted up to 7 days.

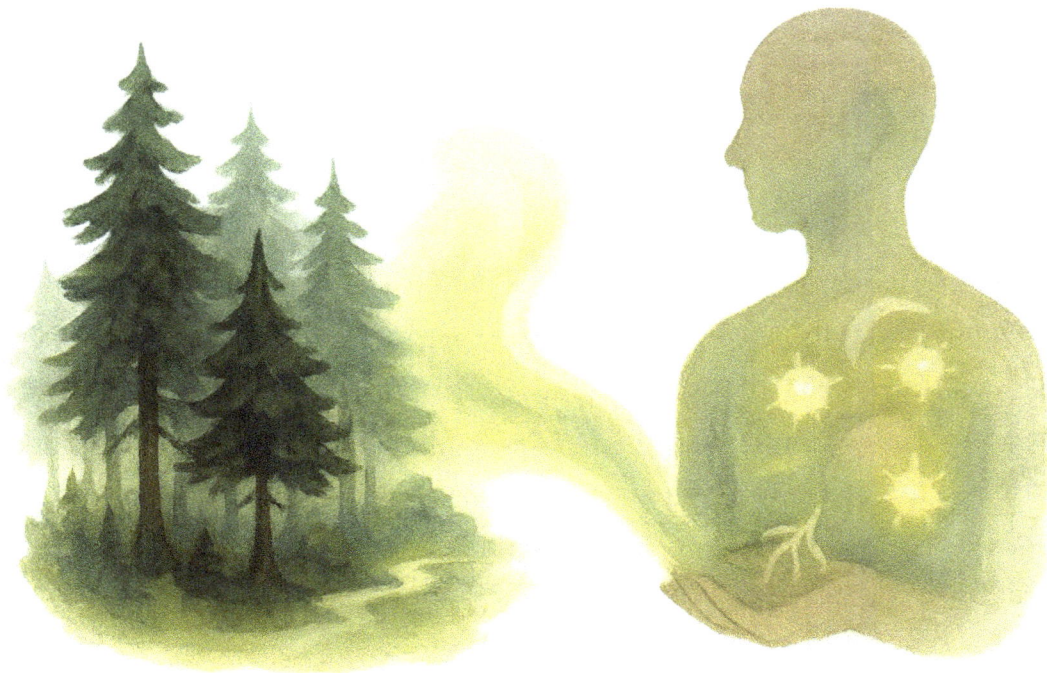

CARDIOVASCULAR & RESPIRATORY HEALTH

Fact: Forest time lowers blood pressure, steadies heart rate, and improves lung function. Clean, ion-rich air nourishes the respiratory system.

Urban Contrast: People in polluted cities experience higher asthma, hypertension, and stress-related disorders—conditions that forests naturally buffer.

MENTAL HEALTH & COGNITION

Fact: Forest environments increase alpha brain waves—the rhythm linked to relaxation, creativity, and focus.

Clinical Finding: Children with ADHD show better concentration and reduced impulsivity after even short walks in parks and wooded spaces.

MICROBIOME & SOIL CONTACT

Fact: Forest soils are alive with beneficial microbes. One, Mycobacterium vaccae, has been shown to elevate mood and enhance immune balance when humans come into contact with soil.

Implication: Barefoot walking, gardening, or simply sitting close to the earth may help reset the human microbiome—linking mental health to soil health.

Modern neuroscience, immunology, and microbiology now echo what sages, monks, and forest dwellers always knew: trees heal. Every inhalation of pine-scented air, every barefoot step on forest soil, is a biological and spiritual medicine.

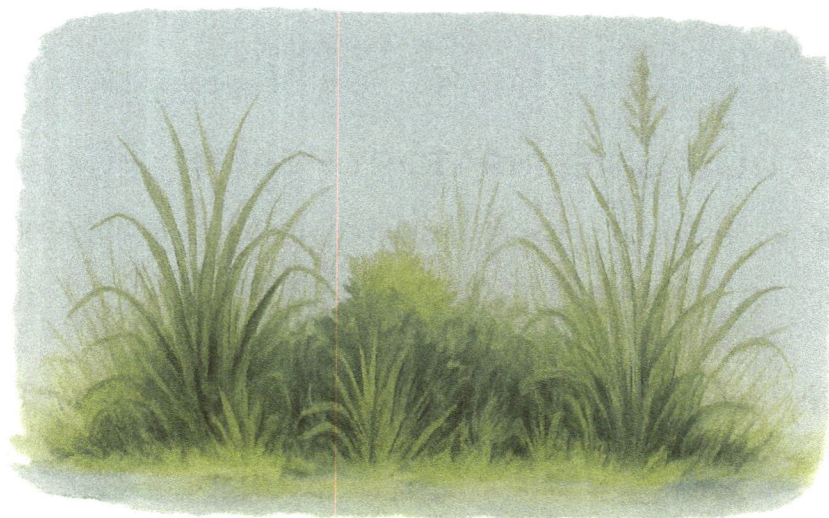

"The tree does not speak, yet it heals.

The shade does not move, yet it transforms.

This is the quiet alchemy of Chhāyā Chikitsā."

INDIAN SPIRITUAL ECOLOGY

Indian spiritual ecology is the unique integration of sacred trees into temple architecture and rituals as a way of subtly giving healing to devotees.

USE OF COMMON SPIRITUAL & NAVAGRAHA TREES IN TEMPLES

1. Peepal Tree (Ficus religiosa)

- Practice: Circumambulation (parikrama) around Peepal is still common.
- Spiritual Reason: Peepal is associated with Lord Vishnu and the Trimurti.
- Healing Reason:
- Emits oxygen even at night → cleanses atmosphere.
- Believed to cleanse aura and strengthen mental clarity.
- Stabilizes prana (life force).

2. Navagraha Vrikshas (Trees of the Nine Planets)

- Many temples still plant trees linked to each graha.
- Example:
    - Arasu (Peepal) → linked to Jupiter.
    - Neem → linked to Mars.
    - Bel (Bilva) → linked to Lord Shiva and Sun.
    - Kadamba → linked to Moon and Krishna bhakti.
- Purpose: Devotees circumambulate these trees to balance planetary energies and receive subtle plant healing.

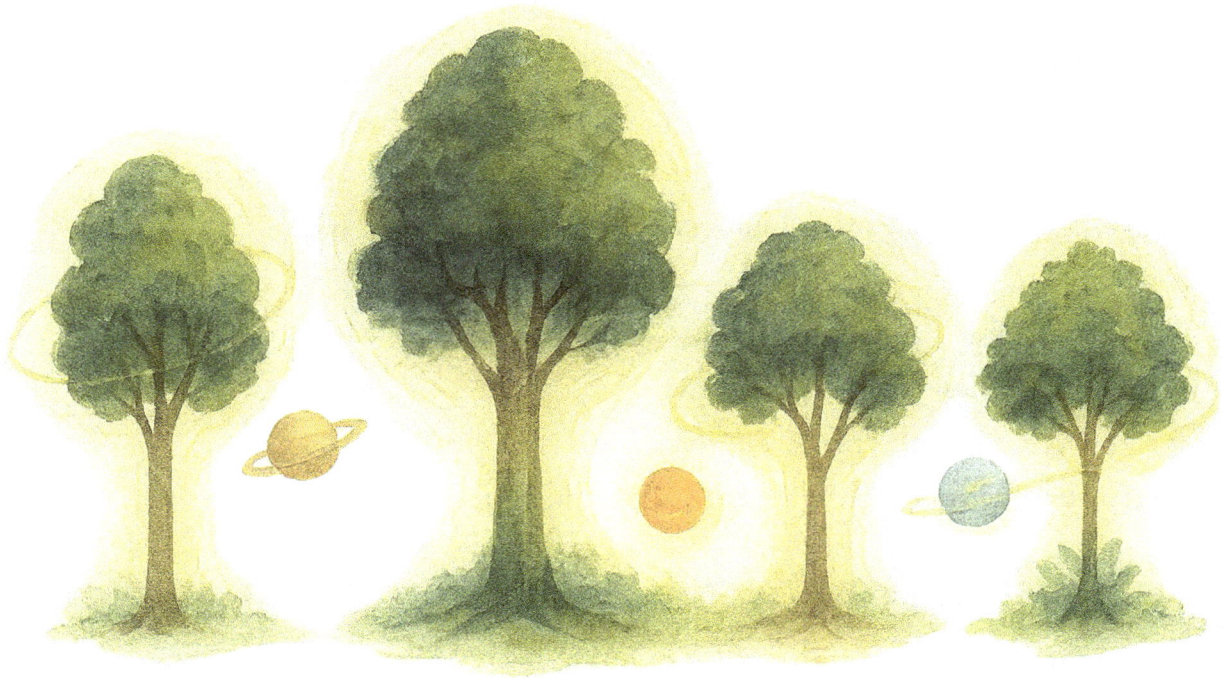

3. Tulsi (Holy Basil)

- Always planted in temple courtyards.
- Spiritual Reason: Beloved of Lord Vishnu.
- Healing Reason: Its volatile oils purify air, reduce stress, and uplift mood.
- Daily puja with Tulsi improves atmosphere and strengthens lungs and immunity.

4. Ashoka Tree (Saraca asoca)

- Found in temple compounds and near Devi shrines.
- Spiritual Reason: Sacred to Kamadeva and Shakti.
- Healing Reason: Symbol of removing sorrow (a-shoka). Just sitting under it brings peace. Its bark is also a powerful gynecological medicine.

5. Banyan Tree (Ficus benghalensis)

- Worshipped as Vat Vriksha.
- Spiritual Reason: Represents Lord Shiva, eternal shelter.
- Healing Reason: Massive aura field → calming effect, grounding energy.
- Couples perform rituals under it for fertility and family harmony.

6. Kadamba (Neolamarckia cadamba)

- Krishna's leela tree in Vrindavan.
- Spiritual Reason: Tree of joy, romance, divine play.
- Healing Reason: Sitting under it uplifts heart and removes melancholy.

The Subtle Wisdom Temple trees are "living healers" → cleansing air, harmonizing prana, balancing grahas, calming the mind.

- By walking around, sitting under, or praying near them, devotees unknowingly receive aura cleansing and physical benefits.
- This is Chhaya Chikitsa in living practice — healing by presence, woven into daily devotion.

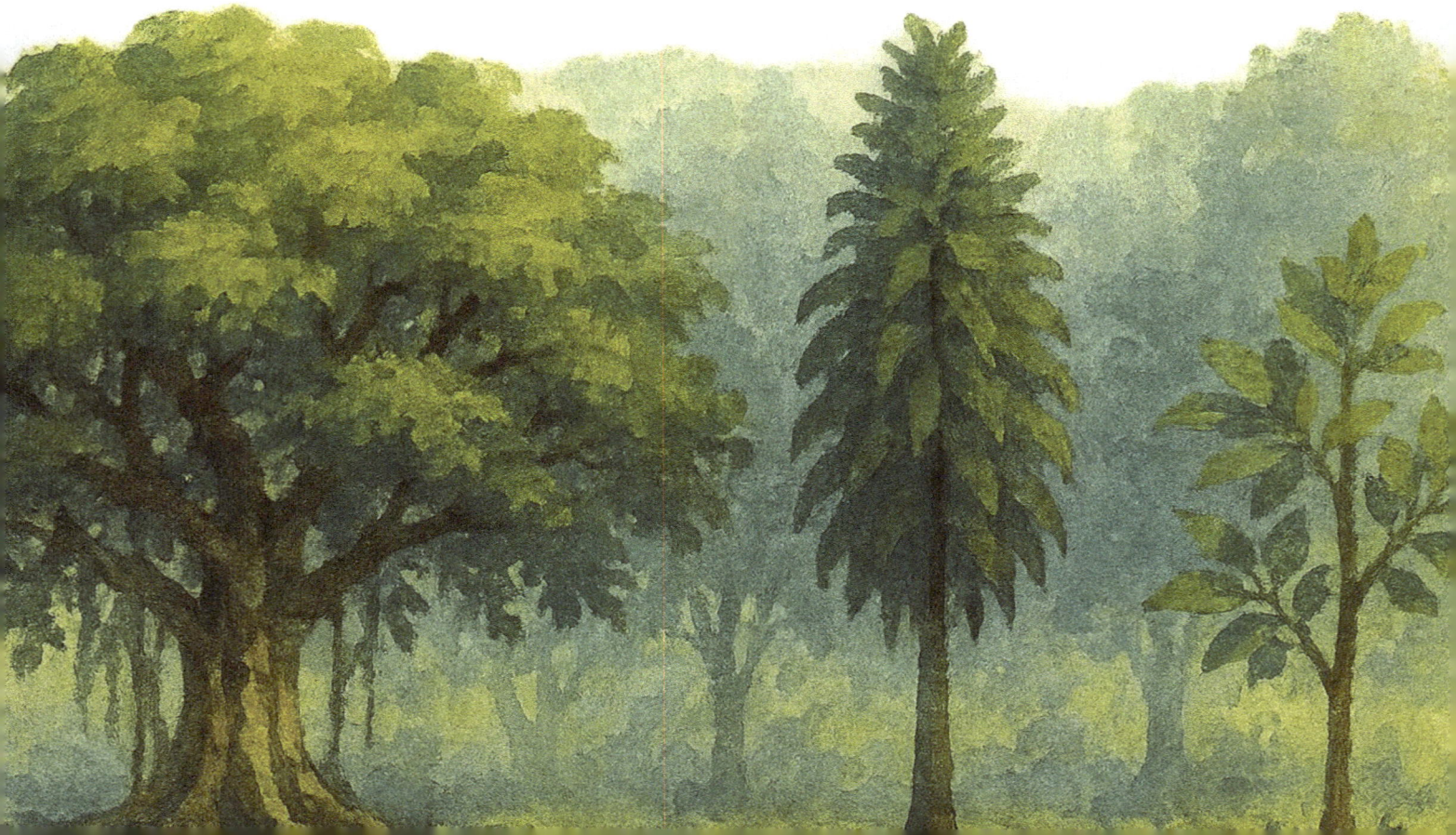

NAVAGRAHA TREES – HEALING & SPIRITUAL CONNECTIONS

Planet (Graha)	Sacred Tree	Temple Practice	Healing / Aura Effect
Surya (Sun)	Arka / Mandar (Calotropis gigantea)	Offer leaves/flowers in Surya temples	Boosts vitality, clarity, removes fatigue; sunlight-like aura strengthening
Chandra (Moon)	Palasha / Kadamba (Butea monosperma / Neolamarckia cadamba)	Circumambulation, offerings on Mondays	Calms the mind, balances emotions, relieves stress, enhances joy
Mangal (Mars)	Khair / Neem (Acacia catechu / Azadirachta indica)	Neem worship on Tuesdays	Purifies blood, antimicrobial atmosphere, strengthens aura against negativity
Budha (Mercury)	Apamarga (Achyranthes aspera)	Used in Budha rituals	Improves intellect, speech, nervous balance
Guru (Jupiter)	Peepal (Ficus religiosa)	Parikrama around Peepal, especially on Thursdays	Enhances wisdom, spiritual growth, cleanses aura, increases prana

Planet (Graha)	Sacred Tree	Temple Practice	Healing / Aura Effect
Shukra (Venus)	Audumbara (Cluster Fig – Ficus racemosa)	Worship under fig trees for fertility & prosperity	Balances reproductive health, fertility, harmonizes relationships
Shani (Saturn)	Shami / Khejri (Prosopis cineraria)	Shami worship during Shani rituals	Grounds energy, relieves karmic burdens, stabilizes nervous system
Rahu	Durva Grass (Cynodon dactylon)	Durva offered to Ganesha, Rahu pacification	Cooling effect, reduces toxins, balances excess energy
Ketu	Kusha Grass (Desmostachya bipinnata)	Used in rituals, asana for meditation	Purifies aura, aids meditation, removes spiritual blockages

Key Insights

- Every graha has a healing tree/plant, linking cosmic balance with ecological healing.
- Temple rituals = subtle therapy → by circumambulating, touching, or sitting under these trees, devotees absorb their aura-cleansing, stress-reducing, prana-enhancing benefits.
- Sacred groves of Navagraha trees (still found in some temples) were ancient "healing gardens."

NAVAGRAHA PLANTS – HEALING, STORIES & DIRECTIONS

1. Surya (Sun) – Arka / Mandar (Calotropis gigantea)

- Qualities: Strong, resilient shrub; its leaves and flowers are used in Surya puja. Latex is medicinal (skin, digestive).
- Metaphysical Story: Arka is said to hold the energy of the Sun God, symbolizing brilliance and vitality. In Surya temples, offering its leaves is said to please Surya and bring clarity.
- Healing Effect: Boosts prana, reduces fatigue, strengthens aura.
- Ideal Direction: East (direction of the Sun).

2. Chandra (Moon) – Kadamba (Neolamarckia cadamba) / Palasha (Butea monosperma)

- Qualities: Soft, fragrant flowers; associated with joy and romance. Its shade is cooling and calming.
- Metaphysical Story: Krishna performed his Rasa Lila under Kadamba trees, linking it with Moon's soothing, emotional, and devotional energy.
- Healing Effect: Calms emotions, relieves stress, balances mind.
- Ideal Direction: North-West (direction of Chandra).

3. Mangal (Mars) – Neem (Azadirachta indica) / Khadira (Acacia catechu)

- Qualities: Bitter leaves, powerful blood purifier, antimicrobial aura.
- Metaphysical Story: Neem is believed to house Goddess Shitala, who cures fevers and infections. Mars' fiery energy is soothed by Neem's cooling nature.
- Healing Effect: Cleans aura, protects from negativity, strengthens immunity.
- Ideal Direction: South (direction of Mars).

4. Budha (Mercury) – Apamarga (Achyranthes aspera)

- Qualities: A humble medicinal herb; roots used in mantras and rituals for Budha.
- Metaphysical Story: Budha (born of Chandra & Tara) is associated with wisdom and speech. Apamarga is used to clear obstacles in chanting and communication.
- Healing Effect: Enhances intellect, clarity, balance of nerves.
- Ideal Direction: North (direction of Mercury).

5. Guru (Jupiter) – Peepal (Ficus religiosa)

- Qualities: Sacred tree, produces oxygen day & night, vast aura field.
- Metaphysical Story: It is said Vishnu resides in Peepal, Shiva in its roots, Brahma in its trunk, hence parikrama is equivalent to worshipping the Trimurti.
- Healing Effect: Expands wisdom, spiritual growth, cleanses aura deeply.
- Ideal Direction: North-East (direction of Jupiter & Ishanya).

6. Shukra (Venus) – Audumbara (Ficus racemosa)

- Qualities: Fig tree, linked with fertility, prosperity, and reproductive health.
- Metaphysical Story: Considered dear to Dattatreya; worship under it blesses with abundance and harmony in relationships.
- Healing Effect: Promotes fertility, balances reproductive energy, prosperity.
- Ideal Direction: South-East (direction of Shukra).

7. Shani (Saturn) – Shami / Khejri (Prosopis cineraria)

- Qualities: Hardy desert tree, survives in harsh conditions, symbol of endurance.
- Metaphysical Story: During exile, Pandavas hid their weapons in a Shami tree; hence it represents protection and karma balancing.
- Healing Effect: Grounds energy, removes karmic burdens, stabilizes mind.
- Ideal Direction: West (direction of Shani).

8. Rahu – Durva Grass (Cynodon dactylon)

- Qualities: Cooling grass, often offered to Lord Ganesha.
- Metaphysical Story: Durva cooled Ganesha's fiery head after he swallowed fire, hence associated with pacifying Rahu's intense energy.
- Healing Effect: Detoxifies, cools body, harmonizes prana.
- Ideal Direction: South-West (direction of Rahu).

9. Ketu – Kusha Grass (Desmostachya bipinnata)

- Qualities: Sacred grass used in Vedic rituals; asana made of Kusha aids meditation.
- Metaphysical Story: Said to have sprung from Lord Vishnu's body during Vamana Avatar. Associated with detachment and moksha.
- Healing Effect: Purifies aura, enhances meditation, removes spiritual blockages.
- Ideal Direction: South-West (near Rahu's direction, but slightly different depending on temple layout).

Summary of Planting Directions

- East → Surya
- North-West → Chandra
- South → Mangal
- North → Budha
- North-East → Guru
- South-East → Shukra
- West → Shani
- South-West → Rahu & Ketu

This way, a Navagraha Vatika (sacred garden of planetary trees) becomes not just symbolic, but an energetic healing mandala

IN THE SHADE OF THE NINE

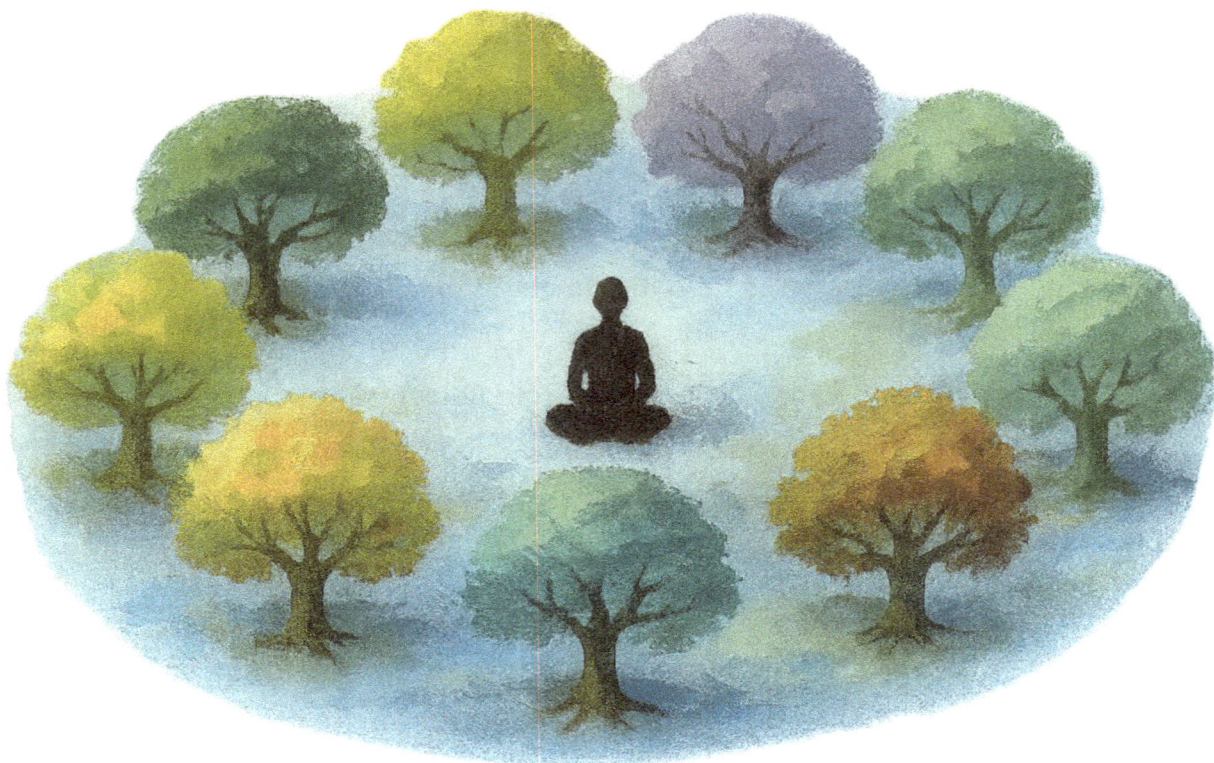

Beneath the sky, where planets shine,
The Navagraha bless through root and vine.
Each tree a guardian, silent, still,
Whispering cures for heart and will.

Surya's Arka, radiant, bright,
Fills our soul with golden light.
In morning shade, fatigue takes flight,
Aura cleansed, the path feels right.

Chandra's Kadamba, tender, sweet,
Where Krishna danced with joy complete.
Its cooling shade dissolves our fears,
Balming hearts, drying tears.

Mangal's Neem, so bitter, strong,
Burns away disease and wrong.
Its shade protects, its breath is pure,
A fiery spirit finds its cure.

Budha's Apamarga, small, profound,
Sharpens thought where minds are bound.
In its presence, clarity flows,
Speech is gentle, wisdom grows.

Guru's Peepal, vast and wise,
Roots in earth, yet touches skies.
Trimurti's home, in shade we find,
Calm for spirit, strength for mind.

Shukra's Audumbara, fig of grace,
Offers love's abundant face.
Couples rest in its embrace,
Fertile joy, a sacred space.

Shani's Shami, austere, deep,
Keeps the vows and karmas we keep.
Its shelter soothes, its strength is slow,
Patience teaches souls to grow.

Rahu's Durva, a humble grass,
Cools the heat where shadows pass.
Laid at Ganesha's feet with care,
Its aura heals the mind's despair.

Ketu's Kusha, slender, true,
Seats the sage in cosmic view.
Its shade dissolves the worldly ties,
Revealing where eternity lies.

Chhaya Chikitsa sings this song:
Sit with trees, you'll find you belong.
Planets above and roots below,
Guide the healing streams that flow.

Love

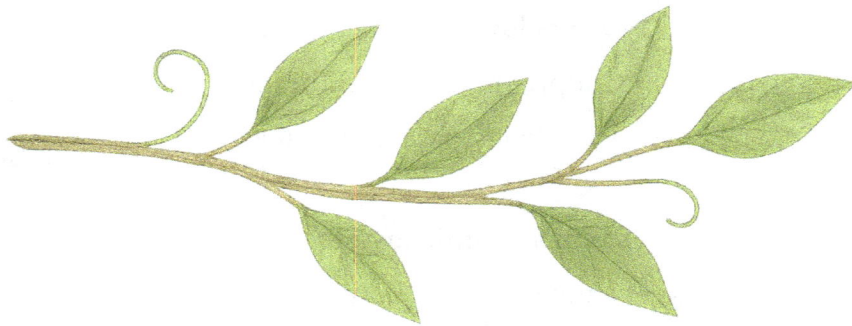

"The tree heals not by giving us
something new, but by returning us to
what we already are—
calm, connected, whole."

HISTORY

SPIRITUAL CONNECTIONS WITH NATURE

Bhagavad Gita & Vrindavan Connection

- Vrindavan forests: The Gita and Krishna leelas describe forests filled with Kadamba, Tulsi, Yamuna groves.

- Tulsi (Holy Basil): Associated with devotion to Krishna; balances mind and immunity.

- Kadamba tree: Krishna played flute under Kadamba trees; symbolizes joy, divine play, and bhakti.

- In the Gita (Chapter 15), Krishna compares the world to the Ashvattha tree (Peepal tree) with roots above and branches below — symbolizing the eternal cosmic order.

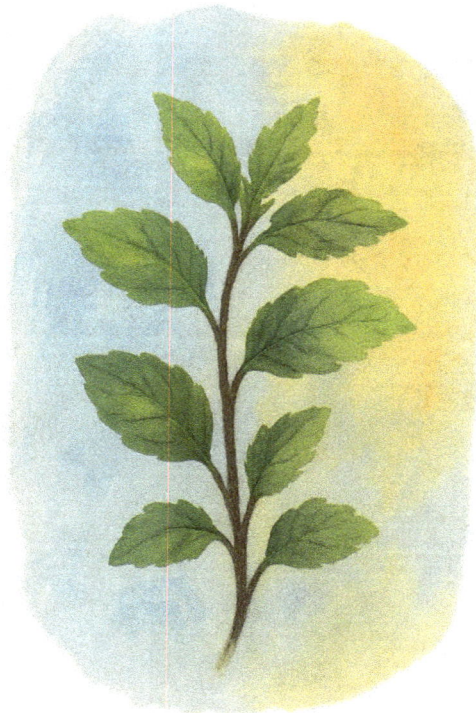

Guru Nanak & Sacred Trees (Sikh Tradition)

- Guru Nanak often meditated under trees (e.g., Beri tree in Sultanpur Lodhi where he attained enlightenment).
- Many gurdwaras still preserve "Guru ke Beri" (sacred jujube/berry trees).
- Symbolism: trees as silent saints, offering shade, fruit, and life without asking in return — embodying seva (selfless service).

Buddha & Sacred Plants

- Bodhi Tree (Peepal, Ficus religiosa): Siddhartha attained enlightenment under the Bodhi tree at Bodh Gaya.
- Symbolism: awakening, shelter of compassion, eternal wisdom.
- In Buddhist texts, forests are recommended for monks for meditation because trees carry natural dharma energy.
- Sala tree: Buddha passed away under twin Sala trees (Parinirvana). Sala represents impermanence and transition.

SHARED THEMES ACROSS TRADITIONS

- Ashoka, Tulsi, Bodhi, Beri, Kadamba → not only plants, but symbols of resilience, purity, and spiritual awakening.
- Forests are described as natural sanctuaries where human suffering is soothed.
- Sacred plants embody both physical healing (Ayurveda) and spiritual nourishment (Dharma, Bhakti, Seva, Shunyata).

SUMMARY

- Ramayana: Ashoka (hope), Jackfruit (abundance), Bilva (Shiva devotion).
- Gita/Vrindavan: Tulsi (devotion), Kadamba (divine play), Peepal (cosmic tree).
- Guru Nanak: Beri tree (seva, silent wisdom).
- Buddha: Bodhi (awakening), Sala (impermanence).

"To know a tree is to
know a medicine.

To sit with a tree is to
meet a friend."

VAASTU

A Vaastu-influenced fragrant garden with white flowers combines sacred geometry, directions, and plant energies to invite peace, purity, and prosperity.

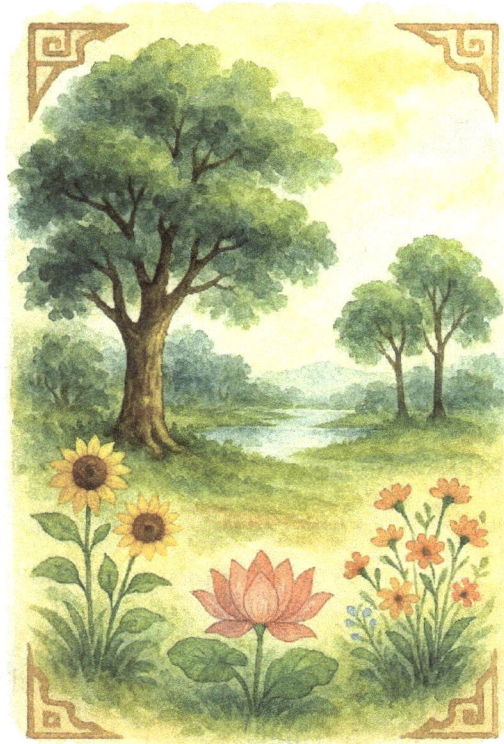

PRINCIPLES OF VAASTU FOR A HEALING WHITE-FLOWER GARDEN

1. Direction & Placement

- North-East (Ishan Kona): Best for white, fragrant, and sacred flowering plants → brings clarity, purity, spiritual upliftment.
- East: Plants with mild fragrance (like jasmine) → enhances vitality and pranic flow with rising sun.
- North: Cooling, soothing, prosperity-bringing plants.
- South & West: Heavier, protective plants (shrubs, shade-giving trees).

2. Why White Flowers?

- Represent Sattva guna (purity, balance, higher consciousness).
- Associated with Moon energy → calmness, fertility, mind stability.
- Traditionally offered in rituals, especially for peace and harmony.

SACRED & FRAGRANT WHITE FLOWERING PLANTS

- Jasmine (Mogra, Chameli, Juhi) → Enhances love, devotion, and moon energy; fragrance calms the mind.
- Parijat (Night-flowering Jasmine, Harsingar) → Mythical flower of heaven; blooms at night, symbol of surrender and divine grace.
- Rajnigandha (Tuberose) → Associated with Venus, brings harmony, marital bliss, and sensual yet serene fragrance.
- Champa/Plumeria (White variety) → Associated with temples; its scent invites positive energy.
- Kadamba (Neolamarckia cadamba, white varieties too) → Krishna's favorite tree; its presence uplifts and heals emotionally.
- Sacred Lotus (White Lotus) → Symbol of purity rising above the mud; linked to Lakshmi and Saraswati.
- Nandyavarta (Crape Jasmine, Tagar) → White pinwheel flowers; balances planetary doshas, often used in rituals.

METAPHYSICAL & RITUAL ASPECTS

- Plant Tulsi in the center → harmonizes energies.
- Watering ritual in the morning with mantra chanting (like Om Somaya Namah for Moon).
- Sitting in the garden during moonlight nights enhances emotional healing and aura cleansing.
- White flowers offered daily at a home shrine or temple channel divine vibrations.

DESIGN CONCEPT

- Lotus pond or water feature in the North-East with floating white lotuses.
- Arched trellis of jasmine in the East.
- Fragrant Kadamba tree (or Champa) in the North for shade and healing aura.
- Rajnigandha rows along walking paths for continuous fragrance.
- Meditation seat under Parijat tree, open to moonlight.

1. East (Indra's direction, Sun, Air element)

- Qualities: Renewal, vitality, spiritual clarity, good health.
- Ideal plants/flowers:
  - White Jasmine (Mogra/Chameli) → purity + Moon-Sun balance.
  - Parijat (Night Jasmine, Harsingar) → blooms in early dawn, sacred offering.
  - Marigold (Orange/Yellow) → Sun energy, removes negativity.
  - Tulsi → spiritual vibration, immunity booster.
- Design tip: Keep space open for morning sunlight; plant low-height fragrant shrubs.

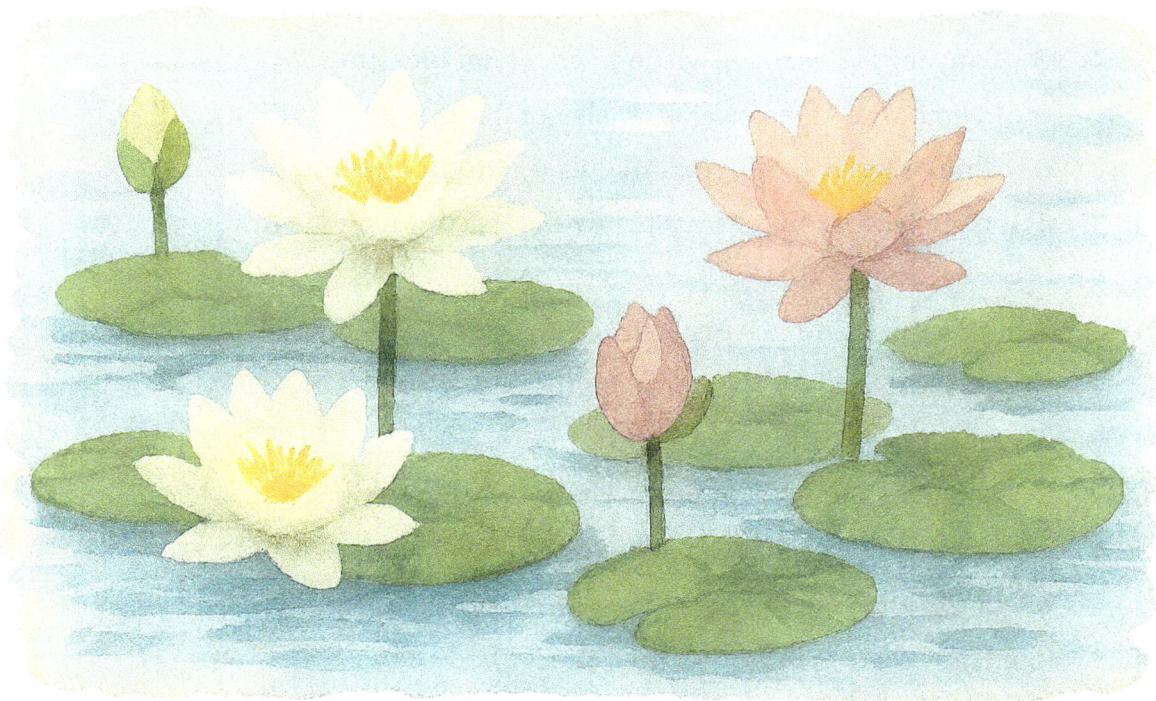

2. South-East (Agni's direction, Fire element, Venus)

- Qualities: Energy, transformation, prosperity.
- Ideal plants/flowers:
  - Rajnigandha (Tuberose) → sensual fragrance, Venus energy.
  - Hibiscus (red) → associated with Agni & Devi worship.
  - Pomegranate plant → fertility & vitality.
- Design tip: Avoid huge trees here; keep vibrant, colorful flowering shrubs.

3. South (Yama's direction, Mars, Fire element)

- Qualities: Strength, discipline, boundaries.
- Ideal plants/trees:
  - Neem tree → purifier, protection.
  - Ashoka tree → emotional healing, auspicious.
  - Red/Orange flowering plants → enhance vitality.
- Design tip: Plant taller trees here for boundary protection.

4. South-West (Nairitya, Rahu/Ketu, Earth element)

- Qualities: Stability, grounding, protection.
- Ideal plants/trees:
  - Banyan tree (Vata) → wisdom, ancestral blessings.
  - Peepal tree (if space allows, else in temple grounds).
  - Thick shrubs like Bougainvillea → natural fencing, security.
- Design tip: Place strong, heavy plants here; avoid water features.

5. West (Varuna's direction, Saturn, Water element)

- Qualities: Patience, nourishment, maturity.
- Ideal plants/trees:
  - Banana plant → abundance, ritual offerings.
  - Champa/Plumeria (white or yellow) → temple fragrance.
  - Lotus pond (small water body) → enhances Varuna's blessings.
- Design tip: Create evening-scented flower beds here.

6. North-West (Vayu's direction, Moon, Air element)

- Qualities: Movement, creativity, harmony.
- Ideal plants/flowers:
  - Tulsi in pots → balance.
  - Jasmine climbers → delicate fragrance for air circulation.
  - Flowering creepers on arches.
- Design tip: Use climbers and plants that sway with wind.

7. North (Kubera's direction, Mercury, Water element)

- Qualities: Wealth, healing, clarity.
- Ideal plants/trees:
  - Sacred Tulsi → spiritual and medicinal.
  - Money Plant or Sacred Basil → prosperity.
  - Kadamba tree → joy, Krishna's divine aura.
- Design tip: Keep a meditation spot in shade here.

8. North-East (Ishan Kona, Jupiter, Water element)

- Qualities: Wisdom, spirituality, peace.
- Ideal plants/flowers:
  - White Lotus pond → sattva, divine purity.
  - Bilva tree → sacred to Shiva, healing aura.
  - White Nandyavarta (Crape Jasmine) → peace and clarity.
- Design tip: Best place for temple corner, small water bodies, meditation nook.

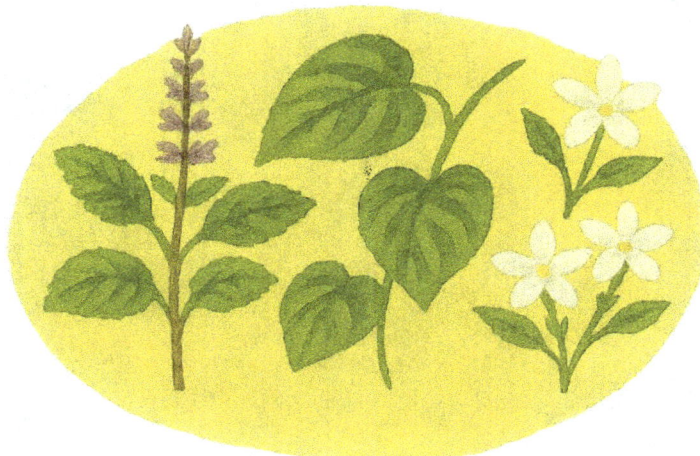

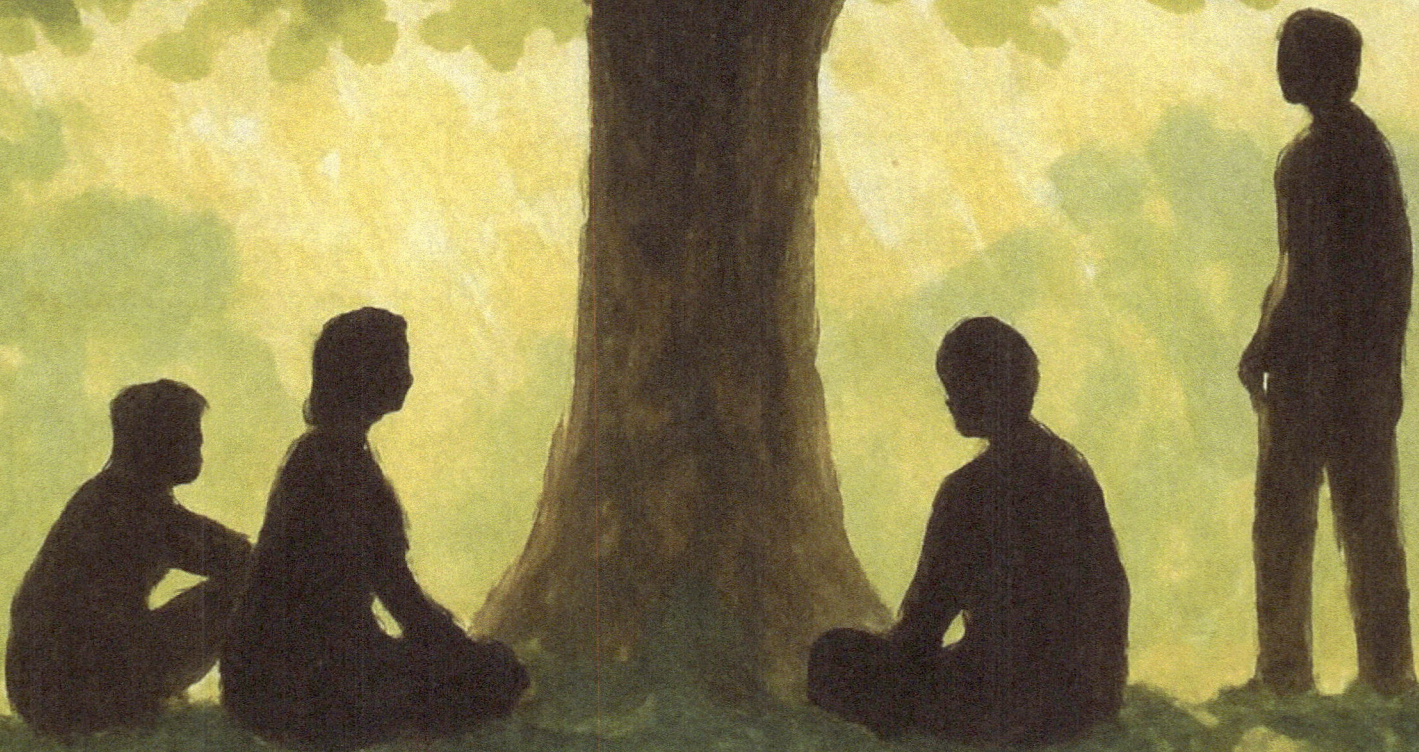

"Plants were our first teachers,
our first medicine, our first prayers."

INDOOR PLANTS

WHY INDOOR PLANTS ARE HEALING COMPANIONS

From ancient homes to modern apartments, plants have always been our silent companions. Indoors, they do more than beautify spaces—they cleanse the air, balance humidity, uplift moods, and radiate subtle energy fields that support well-being. In Ayurveda, Feng Shui, and even NASA studies, indoor plants are celebrated for their ability to filter toxins, produce oxygen, and create harmony.

By choosing the right plants, you invite a living pharmacy and natural energy healer into your home. Each plant carries a story, an energy, and a unique healing vibration that makes your living space more than just walls—it becomes a sanctuary.

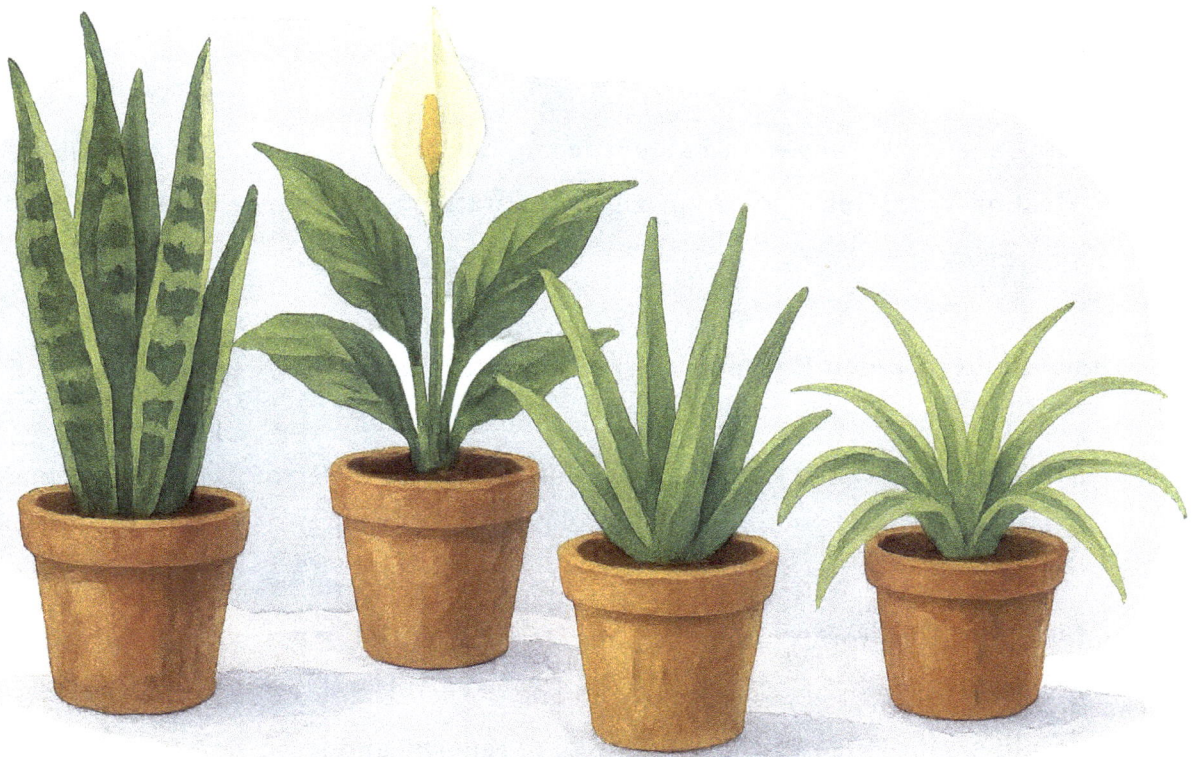

POSITIVE INDOOR PLANTS & THEIR HEALING PROPERTIES

1. Areca Palm (Dypsis lutescens)

- Air Benefits: Excellent natural humidifier; removes xylene and toluene.
- Healing Vibe: Creates a calm, tropical atmosphere; enhances oxygen levels in the home.

2. Snake Plant (Sansevieria trifasciata / Mother-in-Law's Tongue)

- Air Benefits: Converts CO_2 to oxygen at night; removes formaldehyde, benzene, trichloroethylene.
- Healing Vibe: Known as a "bedroom plant" for improving sleep quality and grounding energy.

3. Peace Lily (Spathiphyllum)

- Air Benefits: Filters benzene, formaldehyde, trichloroethylene, and ammonia.
- Healing Vibe: Symbol of purity and peace; absorbs excess mold spores, great for bathrooms.

4. Aloe Vera

- Air Benefits: Cleanses formaldehyde and benzene.
- Healing Vibe: Gel soothes burns, skin irritations, and boosts immunity. A "living pharmacy" plant.

5. Money Plant / Golden Pothos (Epipremnum aureum)

- Air Benefits: Removes formaldehyde, benzene, xylene.
- Healing Vibe: Considered lucky in Vastu/Feng Shui—attracts prosperity and positive energy.

6. Spider Plant (Chlorophytum comosum)

- Air Benefits: Removes carbon monoxide, formaldehyde, and xylene.
- Healing Vibe: Very resilient—symbol of renewal and fresh starts; boosts indoor vitality.

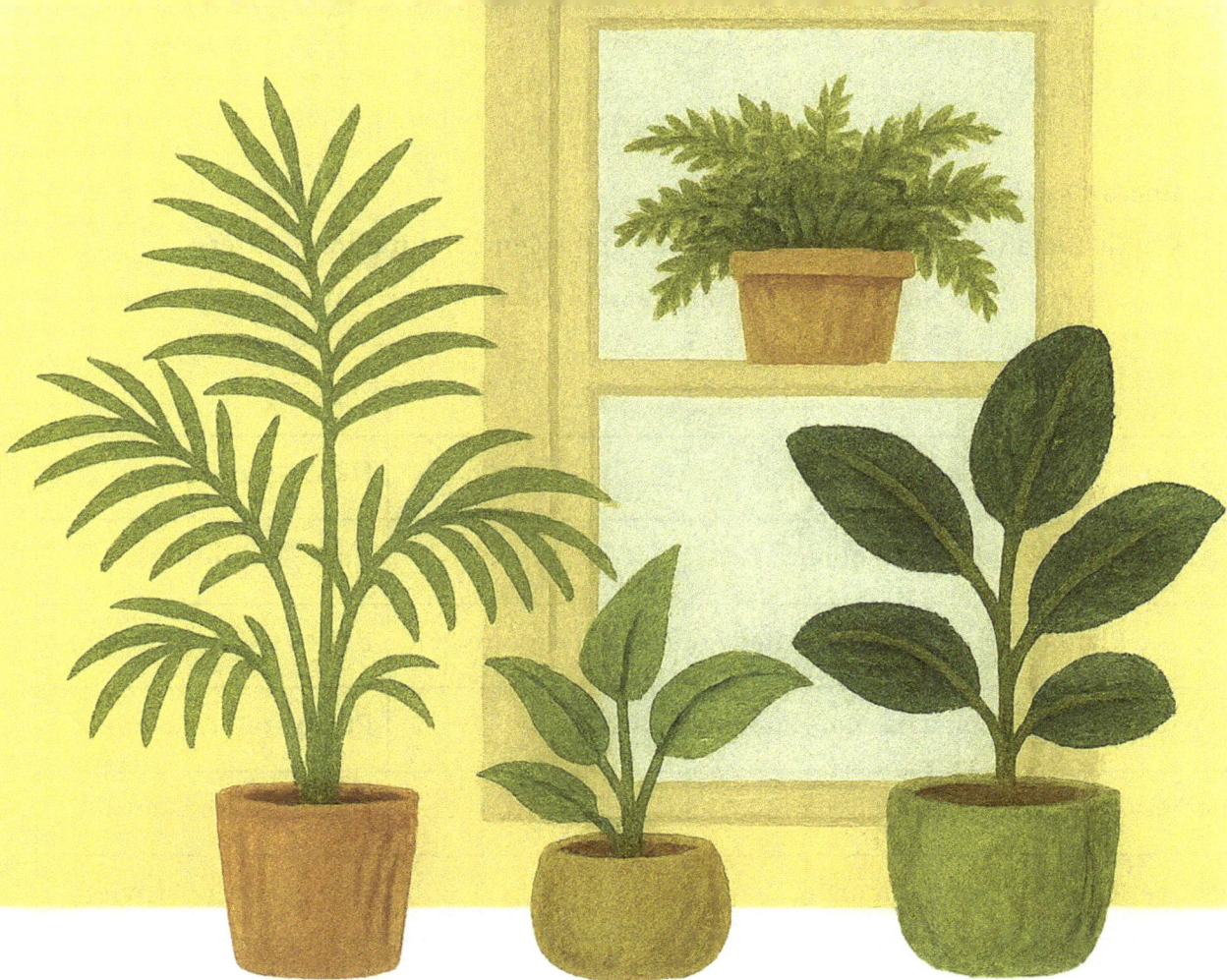

7. Rubber Plant (Ficus elastica)

- Air Benefits: Absorbs airborne toxins like formaldehyde.
- Healing Vibe: Strong, glossy leaves represent abundance and emotional grounding.

8. Bamboo Palm (Chamaedorea seifrizii)

- Air Benefits: Excellent at removing formaldehyde and benzene.
- Healing Vibe: Feng Shui plant—brings harmony, longevity, and good fortune.

9. Tulsi (Holy Basil, Ocimum sanctum)

- Air Benefits: Releases oxygen for 20 hours/day; absorbs carbon dioxide and pollutants.
- Healing Vibe: Sacred Ayurvedic herb—improves immunity, reduces stress, and purifies aura.

10. Boston Fern (*Nephrolepis exaltata*)

- Air Benefits: Removes formaldehyde and xylene; natural humidifier.
- Healing Vibe: Soft, feathery fronds ease mental fatigue and emotional stress.

Plant	Cleanses	Healing Energy
Areca Palm	Xylene, Toluene	Calm, humidifies
Snake Plant	Formaldehyde, Benzene, Trichloroethylene	Better sleep, grounding
Peace Lily	Benzene, Formaldehyde, Ammonia	Purity, reduces mold
Aloe Vera	Formaldehyde, Benzene	Healing skin, soothing
Money Plant	Formaldehyde, Benzene, Xylene	Prosperity, positivity
Spider Plant	CO, Formaldehyde, Xylene	Renewal, fresh starts
Rubber Plant	Formaldehyde	Abundance, grounding
Bamboo Palm	Formaldehyde, Benzene	Harmony, longevity
Tulsi	CO_2, pollutants	Immunity, sacred aura
Boston Fern	Formaldehyde, Xylene	Stress relief

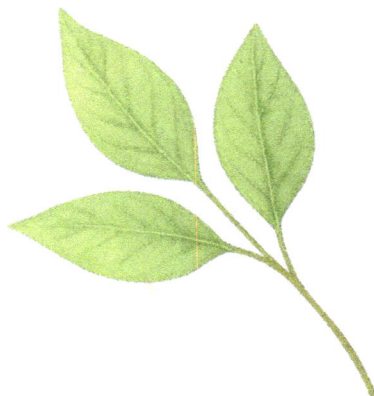

"Like the trees,
may we stay rooted in wisdom
and ever-reaching for the sky."

TRIVANI

The traditional arrangement of planting Neem, Peepal, and Banyan trees together—known as Trivāṇī—is deeply rooted in Indian spiritual and ecological practices. While specific references to this exact trio in ancient scriptures are limited, the individual trees have long been revered in Hinduism, and their collective planting is a manifestation of these traditions.

SPIRITUAL SIGNIFICANCE OF EACH TREE

1. Neem (Azadirachta indica)

- Deity Association: Believed to be associated with Goddess Durga.
- Symbolism: Purity, protection, and the dispelling of negative energies.
- Traditional Use: Leaves and bark are used in various medicinal preparations.

2. Peepal (Ficus religiosa)

- Deity Association: Considered sacred, with Lord Vishnu residing in its roots, Brahma in its trunk, and Shiva in its leaves.
- Symbolism: Longevity, wisdom, and a connection to the divine.
- Traditional Use: Often planted near temples and used in various rituals.

3. Banyan (Ficus benghalensis)

- Deity Association: Represents Lord Vishnu.
- Symbolism: Eternal life, shelter, and community.
- Traditional Use: Commonly found in village centers and used for shade and gathering.

TRIVANI: A COLLECTIVE SPIRITUAL PRACTICE

The practice of planting these three trees together is not explicitly detailed in ancient scriptures but is a part of folk traditions and local customs. It is believed that this arrangement:

- Symbolizes the Unity of the Divine: By planting trees associated with different deities together, it reflects the unity of the divine forces.
- Enhances Spiritual Energy: The combined presence of these trees is thought to amplify spiritual energy in the area.
- Promotes Environmental Harmony: Ecologically, these trees contribute to air purification and provide shelter, aligning with the holistic view of nature in Hindu philosophy.

These traditions have been passed down through generations, often through oral traditions and local customs, rather than being explicitly detailed in ancient scriptures.

While specific references to the Trivānī arrangement are scarce in ancient texts, the individual reverence for these trees is well-documented:

- Peepal Tree: The Peepal tree is considered sacred in Hinduism, with deities residing within it.
- Neem Tree: Neem is revered for its purifying properties and is associated with Goddess Durga.
- Banyan Tree: The Banyan tree is often associated with Lord Vishnu and symbolizes eternal life.

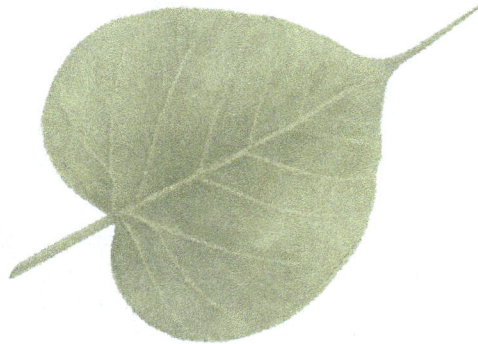

"Before fire and wheel,
before even language—
there was the quiet wisdom
of the forest."

GROUNDING

Grounding, or earthing, is the practice of making direct physical contact with the Earth — soil, grass, sand, or natural water — so that your body can equalize its electrical potential with that of the planet.

- The Earth carries a subtle negative charge, which is naturally abundant with electrons.
- Your body, through exposure to modern electronics and environments, tends to accumulate excess positive charge (a.k.a "dirty electricity" or electromagnetic stress).

DIRTY ELECTRICITY AND MODERN ELECTROMAGNETIC STRESS

- Dirty electricity refers to high-frequency voltage transients produced by devices like Wi-Fi routers, computers, fluorescent lights, smart meters, and power lines.
- These high-frequency spikes can induce extra electrical charge in your body, which may:
- Increase inflammation
- Disrupt nervous system balance
- Disturb sleep and hormonal function

HOW GROUNDING NEUTRALIZES DIRTY ELECTRICITY

1. Direct Connection
- By standing barefoot on grass, soil, or sand, or sitting with your back to the Earth (like in Chhāyā Chikitsā), your body becomes electrically connected to Earth.
- Excess positive charge "flows out" into the Earth, while free electrons from the Earth flow in, neutralizing oxidative stress.

2. Flow of Electrons

- Electrons are antioxidants at a subtle level.
- They reduce free radical activity, calm inflammatory processes, and help the nervous system stabilize.

3. Psychophysiological Benefits

- Heart rate variability improves (better parasympathetic activity).
- Mental clarity, emotional calm, and sleep quality improve.
- The body is literally "discharging" stress and reconnecting to natural rhythms.

THE MOTHER EARTH CONNECTION

- Think of the Earth as a giant grounding pad: it naturally absorbs excess charges that your body doesn't need.
- Ancient practices like sitting under trees (Chhāyā Chikitsā), lying on the ground during forest therapy, or meditating barefoot were practical ways to let the Earth absorb unwanted electrical energy while restoring natural balance.
- This is why humans often feel "recharged" or "lighter" after spending time in nature — it's literally electrical and energetic detoxification.

In short: The secret of grounding may indeed be one of nature's most profound healers. By connecting directly with the Earth, your body discharges unnecessary electromagnetic noise while absorbing restorative energy, bringing physical, mental, and subtle balance — essentially letting Mother Earth do the work that our busy, tech-heavy lives block.

"We returned, weary and wired,
and found the trees still waiting—
with open arms."

GRATITUDE

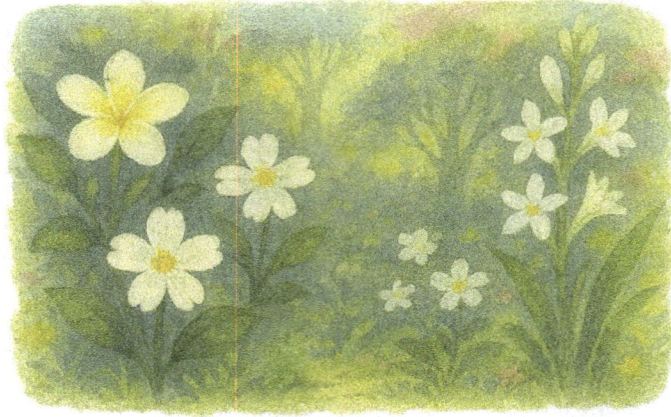

STEPPING INTO NATURE FOR WELLBEING

Holistic health to me
is more than absence of disease—
it is the quiet rhythm of body, mind, and soul
dancing in harmony with Nature's breeze.

It is waking with the sun,
breathing with awareness,
eating with gratitude,
and sleeping with peace.

It is the balance of the five elements—
Earth in my strength,
Water in my flow,
Fire in my passion,
Air in my freedom,
Ether in my silence.

It is listening not only to symptoms
but to the whispers beneath them—
the unheard grief in the hips,
the unspoken burdens on the shoulders,
the tight chest of unshed tears.

It is knowing that food is rasa,
medicine, memory, and mood—
that a banana can soothe,
tulsi can uplift,
and turmeric can heal
not just the body, but the story it holds.

It is trusting that the moon's pull
shapes my emotions,
that my womb is wise,
and that rest is holy.

It is chanting mantras that realign,
touching marma points that awaken,
and honoring the subtle winds of prana
as sacred messengers.

Holistic health to me
is the remembering—
that I am not a machine to be fixed,
but a garden to be nourished,
a temple to be honored,
a mystery to be lived.

The body is not a problem to be solved, but a messenger to be understood.

This belief shapes my approach to health in every way.

I see symptoms not as enemies, but as sacred signals—
the body's intuitive way of asking for balance, attention, or rest.
Rather than suppressing, I listen.
Rather than rushing, I pause.
I ask, "What is this pain trying to say?"
"What emotion lives beneath this tension?"

I believe healing happens when we treat the whole person—
not just the illness, but the inner world:
the thoughts we carry,
the food we digest,
the air we breathe,
the emotions we suppress,
and the spiritual connection we either nourish or neglect.

Holistic health, to me, means respecting this intricate web—
mind, body, heart, and spirit.
And trusting that when we live in tune with nature, with rhythm,
with awareness and love,
we return to wholeness.

Love

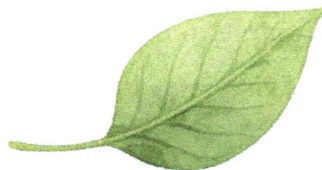

COMBINED PRACTICE GUIDE: CHHĀYĀ CHIKITSĀ + FOREST THERAPY

1. Intention Setting (Sankalpa)

- Before entering the grove/forest, pause.
- Place your hand on your heart. Whisper your intention: "May the shade and spirit of the trees cool my mind, balance my emotions, and restore my wholeness."

2. Enter with Reverence

- Walk slowly, as if you are stepping into a temple.
- Bow inwardly to the trees — in Ayurveda, they are Vriksha Devas (tree deities).
- Modern forest therapy calls this "transitioning" — leaving behind daily concerns as you cross into nature's sanctuary.

3. Find Your Tree or Grove

- Let yourself be drawn naturally — maybe to a Peepal, Banyan, Neem, or any tree whose shade feels inviting.
- This is your Chhāyā seat — the sacred shade for today.

4. Sit in the Shade (Chhāyā Dhyāna)

- Sit comfortably with your back to the trunk or beneath the canopy.
- Allow the dappled sunlight and cool shade to fall on your skin and eyes.
- Close your eyes and breathe gently.
- Feel the tree's prāṇa (life energy) flowing into you with each breath.

5. Sensory Awakening (Forest Therapy Practice)

- See: Observe the play of light and shadow on leaves and earth.
- Hear: Listen to birds, wind, rustling leaves — let sounds wash through you.
- Touch: Place your palm on the tree bark, feel its texture and heartbeat.
- Smell: Breathe in the natural scent of wood, soil, and leaves.
- Taste: If safe, sip cool water or a leaf infusion to merge with the forest essence.

6. Cooling the Mind's Fire

- Visualize your mental restlessness, irritation, or fatigue as heat.
- With each exhale, let this heat dissolve into the cool shade.
- With each inhale, draw in freshness, clarity, and calm from the tree's aura.

7. Silent Absorption

- Rest quietly for 15–30 minutes.
- No forcing thoughts, no trying to meditate.
- Let the shade do the healing — like lying in the lap of Mother Nature.

8. Gratitude & Return

- Before leaving, touch the tree (or bow your head slightly).
- Offer gratitude: "You have cooled my mind and nourished my spirit. Thank you."
- Carry the calmness back with you into your day.

This combined practice helps the mind cool, the heart soften, and the soul reconnect. It's as effective for stress, anxiety, and overthinking as it is for deepening spiritual presence.

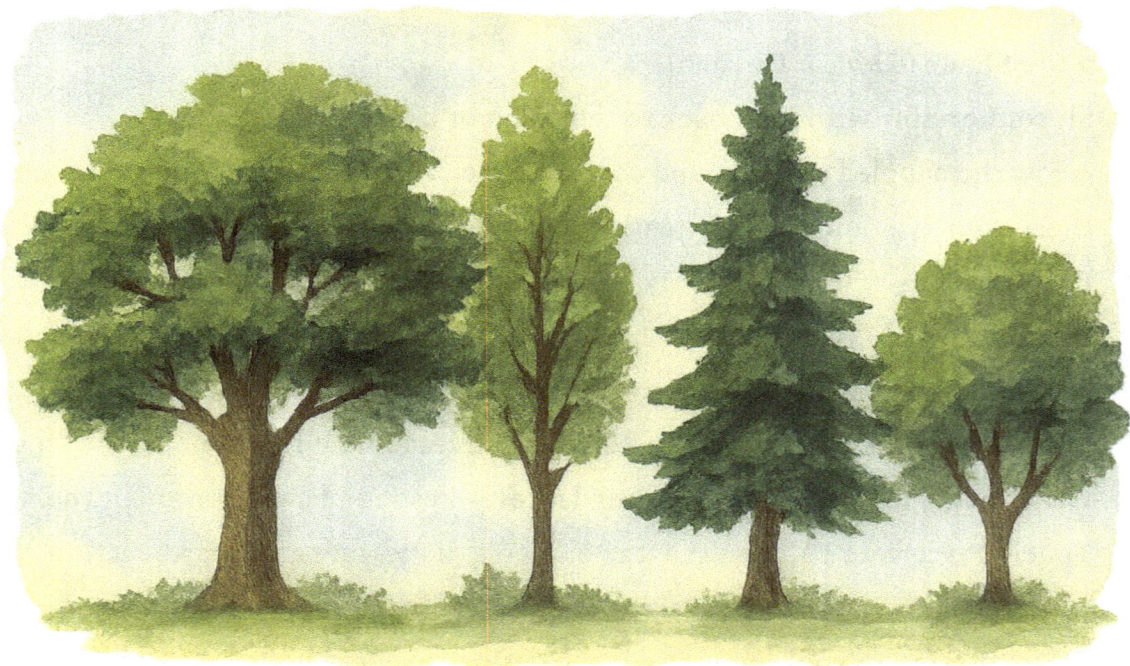

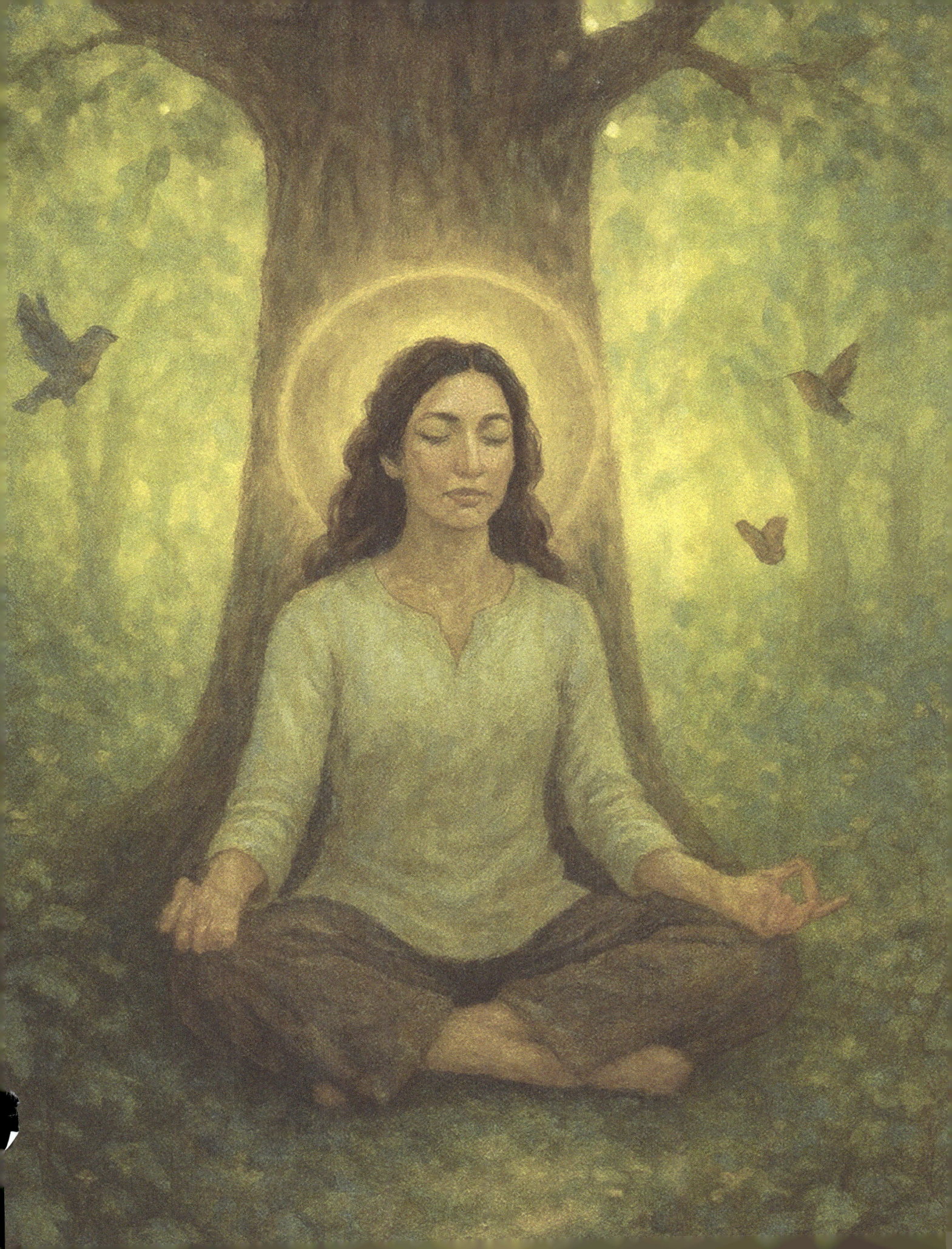

THE SANCTUARY WITHIN – EMBRACING NATURE'S HEALING

In the heart of a forest, the name itself whispers its promise: rest. Rest from work, rest from thoughts, rest from the endless pull of screens and the digital world. Here, under the shade of trees, we are invited to let go — to release the chaotic, unnecessary energies we unknowingly carry. Every leaf, every branch, every subtle vibration of the forest becomes a conduit for healing, grounding, and renewal.

Chhāyā Chikitsā, the ancient Vedic art of shade therapy, meets modern Forest Therapy in this sanctuary, offering a modality so simple it feels revolutionary: you do nothing but be. No medicines, no pills, no yoga, no strenuous practice, no breathing techniques — just presence. The Earth absorbs the excess, chaotic energy; the trees radiate calm, clarity, and a gentle aura of balance. By simply sitting, observing, and connecting, the body releases tension, the mind quiets, and the soul remembers its natural harmony.

This is the power of doing nothing. In that stillness, in that witnessing, we touch Sakshi Bhav, the pure awareness that observes without interference. We experience ascension not by struggle but by surrender — by allowing nature to hold us, restore us, and teach us the rhythm of life that we so often forget.

Imagine a city where green sanctuaries exist on every street corner, in every neighborhood — pockets of forest therapy, living reminders of the Earth's grace. Spaces where children, elders, and workers alike can reconnect with themselves and with the planet. Respecting forests is not just an ecological duty; it is a spiritual act, a gift to our collective consciousness.

This is healing in its purest form: effortless, timeless, profound. You don't have to do anything but show up, be present, and let the forest, the shade, and the Earth do the work. Nature's medicine asks nothing from us — only that we pause, that we witness, and that we allow.

In the embrace of trees, under the gentle play of light and shadow, we remember what was always true: healing is simple, presence is power, and doing nothing can be everything.

Step Into Yourself.

Rest. Release. Recharge.

No pills. No exercises. No routines. Just you, the shade, and the Earth.

Let the forest absorb your chaos. Let the trees radiate calm. Let the soil ground your energy. In this simple act of being, your mind clears, your body relaxes, and your soul remembers its natural balance.

Imagine green sanctuaries in every city, every neighborhood — places to pause, breathe, and reconnect. Respect the forest. Protect it. Honor it.

Do nothing. Witness everything. Heal effortlessly.

The Mother Nature is waiting. Are you ready to just be?

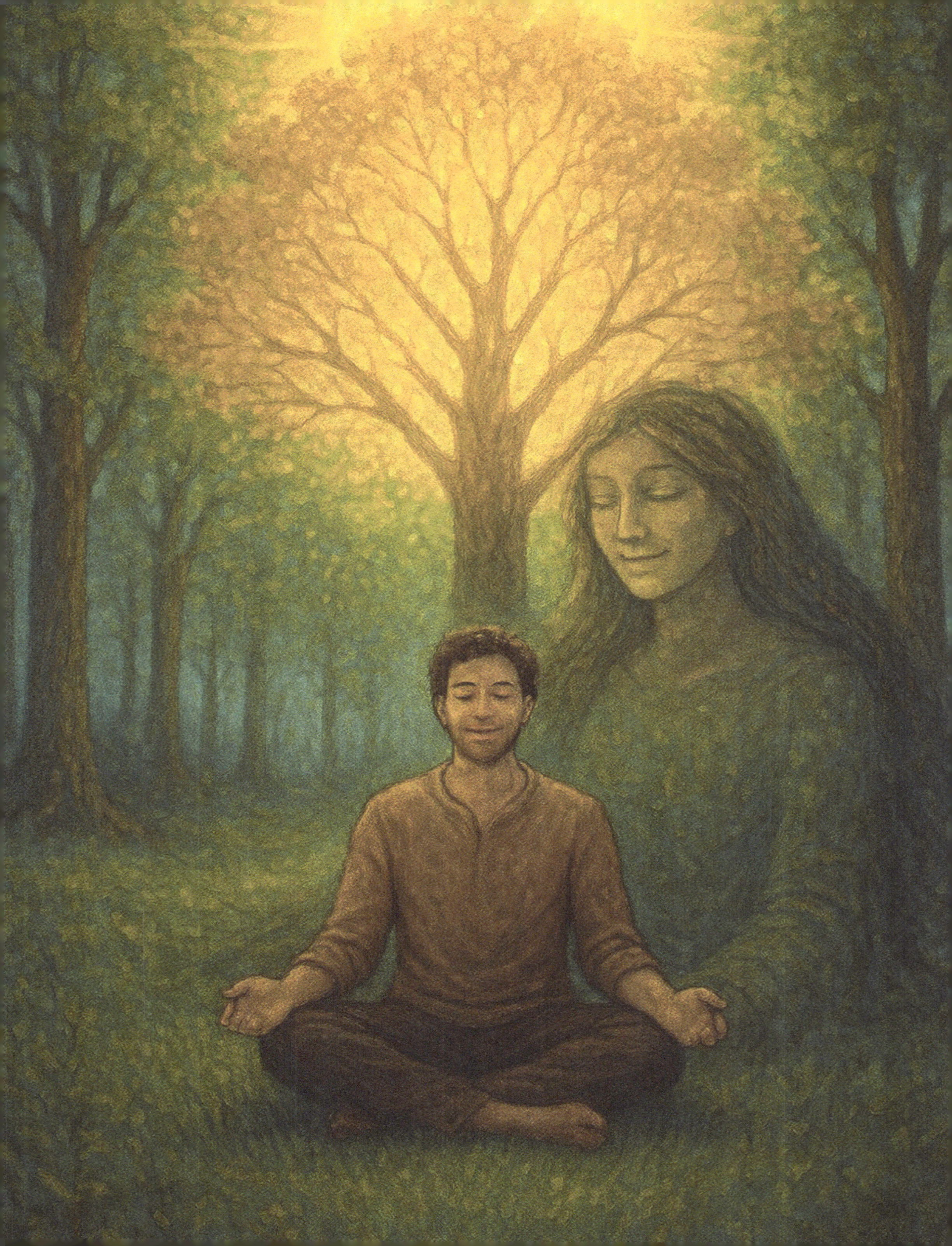

"Prakriti, the eternal Mother,
already holds within her
the rhythm of balance and healing.

Wellness is not something we chase—
it is our original nature.

When we stop resisting
and begin to flow with her wisdom
which is expressed by her seasons,
her intelligence restores harmony
to body, mind, and spirit.

To embrace Prakriti is to return home
to wholeness."

"Trees are poems that the earth writes upon the sky."

- Khalil Gibran

"Trees are the earth's endless effort
to speak to the listening heaven."

- Rabindranath Tagore

_____

_____

_____

_____

_____

_____

_____

_____

_____

"The clearest way into the Universe
is through a forest wilderness."

- John Muir

"When we plant trees, we plant the seeds of peace and hope."

- Wangari Maathai

"A tree is beautiful, but what's more, it has a right to life;
like water, the sun and the stars, it is essential.
Life on earth is inconceivable without trees."

- Mehmet Murat Ildan

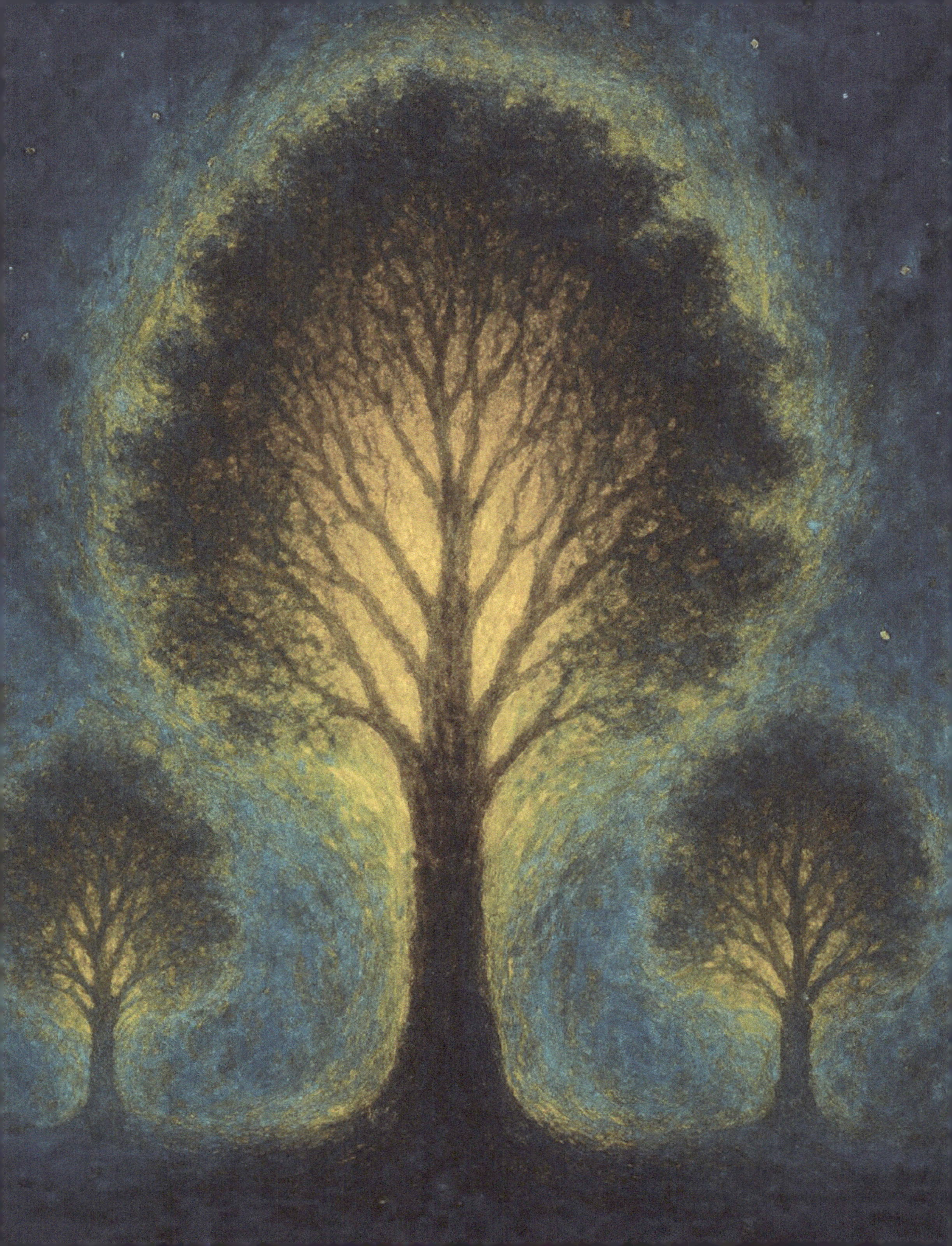

ECHOES OF WISDOM

"The tree which moves some to tears of joy is in the eyes of others only a green thing
that stands in the way."

- William Blake

❁

"For me, trees have always been the most penetrating preachers."

- Herman Hesse

❁

"The creation of a thousand forests is in one acorn."

- Ralph Waldo Emerson

❁

"Even if I knew that tomorrow the world would go to pieces,
I would still plant my apple tree."

- Martin Luther

❁

"The best time to plant a tree was 20 years ago.
The second-best time is now."

- Chinese Proverb

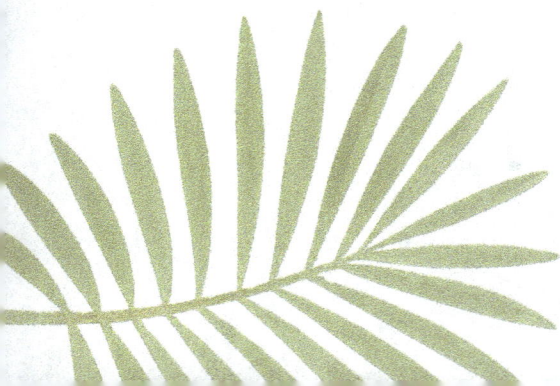

❁

"I took a walk in the woods and came out taller than the trees."

- Henry David Thoreau

❀

"The best friend on earth of man is the tree:
when we use the tree respectfully and economically,
we have one of the greatest resources of the earth."

- Frank Lloyd Wright

❀

"Try to accept the changing seasons of your heart, even as you have always accepted the
changing seasons that pass over your fields."

- Rumi

❀

"The trees will tell their secrets to those that tune in."

- Terri Guillemets

❀

"There is a pleasure in the pathless woods,
there is a rapture on the lonely shore...
I love not man the less, but Nature more."

- Lord Byron

❀

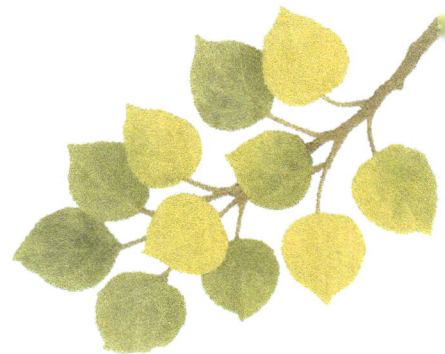

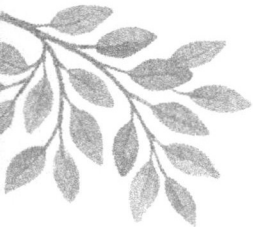

"I think that I shall never see a poem as lovely as a tree."

- Joyce Kilmer

✿

"Trees have a secret life that is only known
to the woods themselves."

- George Nakashima

✿

"Colors are the smiles of nature.
Trees are the laughter of the earth."

- Leigh Hunt

✿

"The woods are full of fairies; the trees are all alive.
The river overflows with them, see how they dip and dive."

- Enid Blyton

✿

"Each time a man looks into the world, he is looking into the forest."

- Karen Joy Fowler

✿

"Whatever befalls the earth befalls the sons of the earth.
If men spit upon the ground, they spit upon themselves."

- Chief Seattle

"If you remember me, then I don't care if everyone else forgets. Memories warm you up from the inside. But they also tear you apart. Like the wind in the trees."

- Haruki Murakami

"He who plants a tree plants a hope."

- Lucy Larcom

"A tree is known by its fruit, a man by his deeds.
A good deed is never lost."

- Dante Alighieri

"I want to do with you what spring does with the cherry trees."

- Pablo Neruda

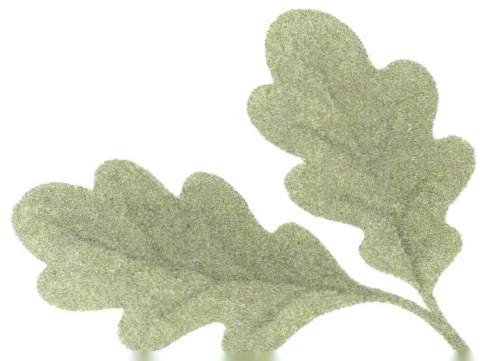

"For my part, I know nothing with any certainty, but the sight of the stars makes me dream. And the sight of trees makes me calm."

- Vincent Van Gogh

"I felt my lungs inflate with the onrush of scenery—air, mountains, trees, people. I thought, this is what it is to be happy."

- Sylvia Plath

"The trees and the grasses and all things growing or living in the land belong each to themselves."

- J.R.R. Tolkien

"To describe my mother would be to write about a hurricane in its perfect power. Or the climbing, falling colors of a rainbow. Or the steady strength of a tree."

- Maya Angelou

"The surface of the Earth is the shore of the cosmic ocean.
On this shore, trees are the children of starlight."

- Carl Sagan

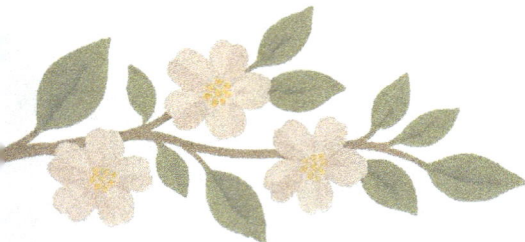

"When we build, let us think that we build forever. Let it not be for present delight nor for present use alone. Let it be such work as our descendants will thank us for; and let us think, as we lay stone on stone, that a time is to come when these stones will be held sacred because our hands have touched them. The same is true with trees."

- John Ruskin

✿

"It is the time you have wasted for your rose that makes your rose so important. And for trees, it is the love you give them that makes them grow."

- Antoine de Saint-Exupéry

✿

"We do not inherit the earth from our ancestors; we borrow it from our children."

- Native American Proverb

✿

"He that plants trees loves others besides himself."

- Thomas Fuller

✿

"The best friend of nature is the man who plants trees."

- Aristotle

✿

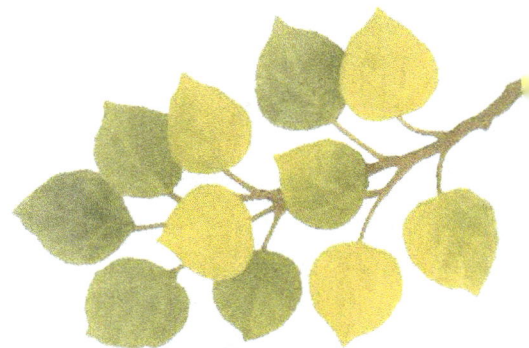

"We cannot live only for ourselves.
A thousand fibers connect us with our fellow men;
and among those fibers are the roots of trees."

- Herman Melville

❀

"Listen to the trees as they sway in the wind.
Their leaves are telling secrets."

- Elizabeth Barrett Browning

❀

"Except during the nine months before he draws his first breath,
no man manages his affairs as well as a tree does."

- George Bernard Shaw

❀

"The old Lakota was wise. He knew that a man's heart,
away from nature, becomes hard. He knew that lack of respect
for growing, living things soon led to lack of respect for humans too."

- Chief Luther Standing Bear

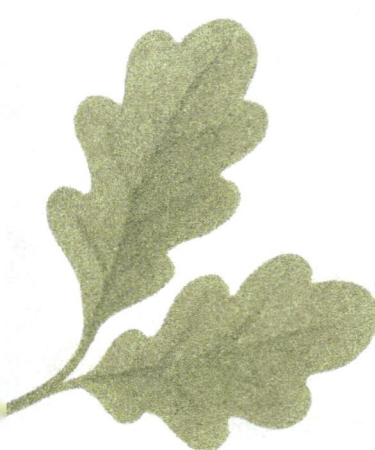

❀

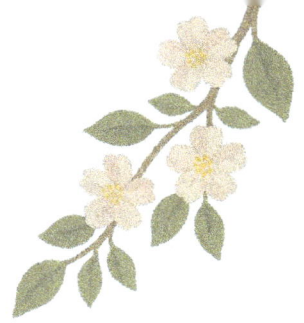

"If you reveal your secrets to the wind,
you should not blame the wind
for revealing them to the trees."

- Kahlil Gibran

❀

"We are living on this planet as if we had another one to go to.
The trees remind us we do not."

- Terri Swearingen

❀

"Everything in nature invites us constantly to be what we are."

- Gretel Ehrlich

❀

"There is in all things a pattern that is part of our universe.
It is in the branches of the trees and the roots of the earth."

- Euripides

❀

"I perhaps owe having become a painter to flowers and trees."

- Claude Monet

❀

"The true meaning of life is to plant trees under whose shade
you do not expect to sit."

- Mark Twain

❀

"A tree that is unbending is easily broken."

- Lao Tzu

❀

"Look deep into nature, and then you will
understand everything better."

- Albert Einstein

❀

"Trees are the effort of the earth to speak to the listening heaven."

- Victor Hugo

❀

"Though a tree grows so high, the falling leaves return to the root."

- Japanese Proverb

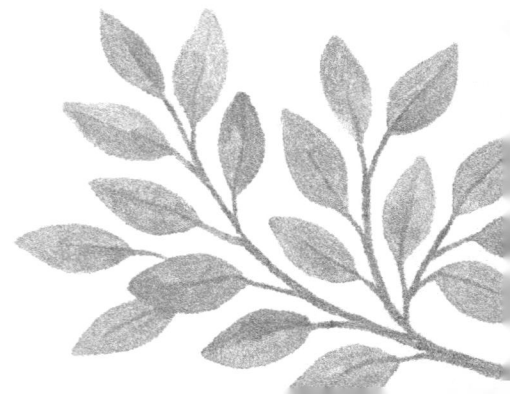

❀

PROFOUND STATEMENTS ON TREES & NATURE
BY SRI SATHYA SAI BABA

"The tree can teach you forbearance and tolerance.
It offers shade to all, irrespective of age,
sex or religion, nationality or status.
It helps with fruit and shade even to the foe
who lays his axe on its trunk!"

❀

"Plant the seeds of Love in your hearts.
Let them grow into trees of Service
and shower the sweet fruit of Ananda.
Share the Ananda with all.
That is the proper way to celebrate the Birthday."

❀

"God is the Seed;
The Universe is the Tree,
Impulses and passions are the branches,
Intelligence is the flower,
Pure Consciousness is the fruit,
Love is the sweetness in the fruit."

❀

"Trees provide the timber for constructing houses and also firewood for domestic use…
Among animate beings, every creature …
is of assistance to man in one way or another. …
Nature's role is to help man, the crowning achievement of the evolutionary process, to
realize the Divinity immanent in creation."

❀

"Trees teach the lesson of sacrifice in that they not only bear fruits while they are alive,
but also give away their body to be used as firewood once the life goes out of them."

❀

"A tree can spread its branches wide. Its branches can bring forth blossoms which yield
fruit, but only when the roots are fed with water. Instead, if the water is poured on
branches, fruits or flowers, can the tree grow and spread? Society has as its root of
peace and prosperity, the virtues of devotion and dedication."

❀

"Man should treat nature with reverence.
He has no right to talk of conquering nature or exploiting
the forces of nature. He must proceed to visualize God in nature."

❀

TO GO WITHIN

To go within, you truly don't need anything.
Self-realization is not an achievement —
it is our most natural state, our original rhythm.
Yet we have made it seem distant,
hidden behind practices, goals, and complexities of the mind.

In truth, going within is a return — not a journey.
It begins when we stop striving and simply become present.

Chaya Chikitsa, the therapy of the shadow and rest,
invites us to do almost nothing —
to lie under a tree, to sit by the mountain,
to let the breeze touch our skin,
to melt into nature's slow heartbeat.

When you rest in your own shadow,
when you allow stillness to hold you,
you begin to sense that silence is not emptiness —
it is fullness, peace, and the doorway to your inner light.

So go — not to achieve, but to receive.
Not to seek, but to see.
Go to the forest, the river, or the quiet mountain that calls you —
and just be.
That is all the medicine the soul ever needed.

Love and Light
Rev. Dr. Gauri M Relan

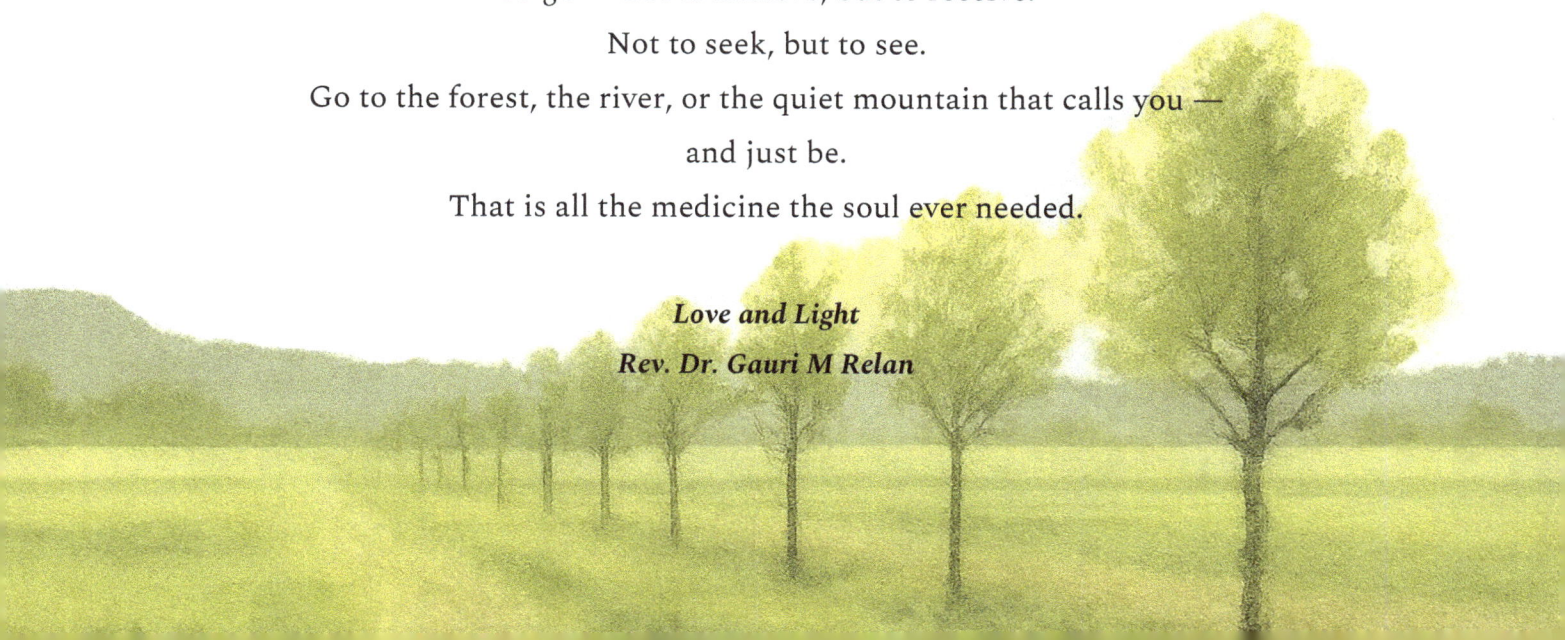

ABOUT THE AUTHOR

Rev. Dr. Gauri M Relan is an accomplished Holistic Healer, specializing in Natural, Vedic, and Metaphysical healing and has been healing since 1995 based on ancient Vedic philosophy of healing at Physical, Emotional, Mental and Spiritual level, so that there is total rejuvenation of physical health, emotional happiness with positive set of minds for one to finally grow spiritually. Dr. Gauri learnt various forms of Meditation and Energy healing techniques from Great Grand Masters of Reiki and Melchizedek and is a certified REIKI Master in Dr. Usui Mikao system.

Dr. Gauri did her Masters M.Sc (Botany), M.Phil (Wood Sciences & Forestry) from Himachal University Shimla, INDIA, 1992 and Ph.D from UMS, California, USA, plus numerous certification in Complimentary, Alternative & Integrative medicine from Harvard Medical School, Stanford and NIH- NCCAM (National Institutes of health - National Center for Complementary and Alternative Medicine) USA Gov. Dr Gauri was ordained as REVEREND by Wisdom of The Heart Church, California, USA, in the year 2010. She is a certified Yoga Instructor from SVYASA University, Bangalore, a certified NLP Master Practitioner & Numerologist from American university of NLP and Certified Hypnotist from American Alliance of Hypnotists.

Dr. Gauri is co-founder of Wellbeen Aeons Research Center Pvt. Ltd (www.wellbeen.com). She has authored many e-books on Apple iBooks and Amazon Kindle, APPS and many courses on UDEMY on Metaphysical self-help techniques. She has conducted numerous workshops in many corporate, many welfare clubs & societies, various schools and colleges in Bangalore. She conducts classes on YOGA, Reiki, Tarot and various Vedic and metaphysical methodologies.

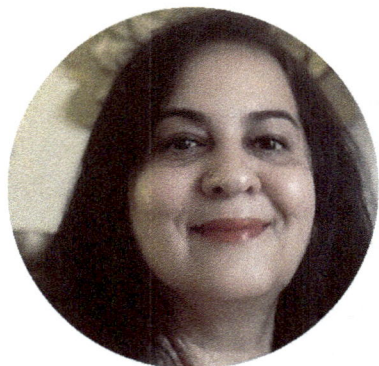

ABOUT THE DESIGNER

Sanyukta Shanbhag is a creative designer who transforms ideas into engaging visual experiences, blending layouts, color, and modern digital tools to make complex concepts feel intuitive and inviting.

Inspired by art, nature, and everyday details, she crafts visuals that spark curiosity, connect meaningfully with audiences, and leave a lasting impression.

❁ ❁ ❁ ❁ ❁

DISCLAIMER

The contents of this book are for informational purposes only and do not render any medical or psychological advice, opinion, diagnosis, or treatment. The information provided should not be used for diagnosing or treating a health problem or disease and no attempt is being made to provide diagnosis, care, treatment, or rehabilitation of individuals, or apply medical, mental health or human development principles to provide diagnosing, treating, operating, or prescribing for any human disease, pain, injury, deformity, or physical condition.

The statements and the products have not been evaluated by FDA and the services and products are not intended to diagnose, treat, cure or prevent any disease or medical condition. The information contained herein is not intended to replace a one-on-one relationship with a doctor or qualified health professional. Any techniques address only the underlying spiritual issues to address energetic blockages that may have an impact on wellness and energetic balance, facilitating the body's natural ability to bring itself to homeostasis, which may have an impact on health and well-being. This book is not a substitute for professional health care. If you have or suspect you may have a medical or psychological problem, you should consult your appropriate health care provider. Never disregard professional medical advice or delay in seeking it because of something you have read on this website. Links on this website are provided only as an informational resource, and it should not be implied that we recommend, endorse or approve of any of the content at the linked sites, nor are we responsible for their availability, accuracy or content. Any review or other matter that could be regarded as a testimonial or endorsement does not constitute a guarantee, warranty, or prediction regarding the outcome of any consultation. The testimonials on this website represent the anecdotal experience of individual consumers. Individual experiences are not a substitute for scientific research.

www.ingramcontent.com/pod-product-compliance
Lightning Source LLC
Chambersburg PA
CBHW080207300326
41934CB00038B/3403